W9-BEC-272

yoga basics

Yoga

BASICS

**C. Alexander Simpkins, Ph.D.
and Annellen Simpkins, Ph.D.**

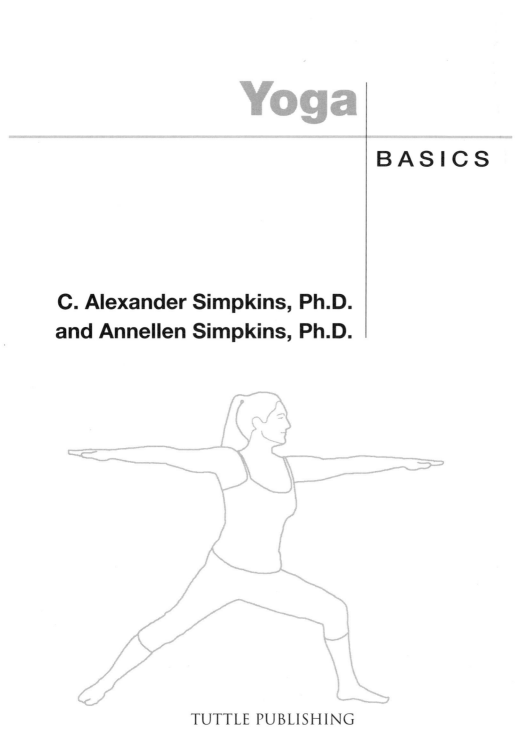

TUTTLE PUBLISHING
Boston · Rutland, Vermont · Tokyo

Please note that the publisher and author(s) of this instructional book are NOT RESPONSIBLE in any manner whatsoever for any injury that may result from practicing the techniques and/or following the instructions given within. Martial arts training can be dangerous—both to you and to others—if not practiced safely. If you're in doubt as to how to proceed or whether your practice is safe, consult with a trained martial arts teacher before beginning. Since the physical activities described herein may be too strenuous in nature for some readers, it is also essential that a physician be consulted prior to training.

First published in the United States in 2003 by Tuttle Publishing, an imprint of Periplus Editions (HK) Ltd., with editorial offices at 153 Milk Street, Boston, Massachusetts 02109.

Copyright © 2003 Tuttle Publishing

All rights reserved. No part of this publication may be reproduced or utilized in any form or by any means, electronic or mechanical, including photocopying, recording, or by any information storage and retrieval system, without prior written permission from Tuttle Publishing.

Library of Congress Cataloging-in-Publication data

Simpkins, C. Alexander
  Yoga basics / C. Alexander Simpkins and Annellen Simpkins.— 1st ed.
    p. cm.
  Includes bibliographical references.
  ISBN 0-8048-3485-7 (pbk.)
    1. Yoga—history. 2. Yoga, Hatha. 3. Physical fitness. I. Simpkins, Annellen M. II. Title
RA781.7.S5572003
613.7'046—dc21   2003054003

Distributed by

North America, Latin America,
and Europe
Tuttle Publishing
Distribution Center
Airport Industrial Park
364 Innovation Drive
North Clarendon, VT 05759-9436
Tel: (802) 773-8930
Fax: (802) 773-6993
Email: info@tuttlepublishing.com

Asia Pacific
Berkeley Books Pte. Ltd.
130 Joo Seng Road
#06-01/03 Olivine Building
Singapore 368357
Tel: (65) 6280-3320
Fax: (65) 6280-6290
Email: inquiries@periplus.com.sg

Japan
Tuttle Publishing
Yaekari Building, 3F
5-4-12 Ōsaki, Shinagawa-ku
Tokyo 141-0032
Tel: (03) 5437-0171
Fax: (03) 5437-0755
Email: tuttle-sales@gol.com

First edition
08 07 06 05 04 03   9 8 7 6 5 4 3 2 1
Printed in the United States of America

table of contents

Part 5: *Making Progress*   169

Acknowledgments

We dedicate this book to our parents, Carmen and
Nathaniel S. Simpkins, Naomi and Herbert L. Minkins,
and to our children, Alura Aguilera and C. Alexander Simpkins Jr.

We wish to thank Alura Aguilera, C. Alexander Simpkins Jr.,
Mary Durham, and Ryan Ferguson for their careful posing of asanas.

preface

YOGA IS MORE than just a form of physical exercise. It is also a deeply philosophical ancient practice that can transform and enhance the quality of life. The many benefits of yoga are revealed by the word itself, which means "to yoke or unify." By practicing yoga, you learn how to unite your mind and body. This oneness begins with the *asanas*, postures that are practiced along with a meditative focus and carefully controlled breathing, or *pranayama*. In time, this combination results in a generally healthier, calmer, and more aware way of being. Mental discipline improves along with physical capacity.

Anyone can do yoga, and people of all ages and physical abilities will easily find their way into the practice by approaching it correctly. This book shows beginners how to practice yoga safely and carefully. More experienced practitioners will find routines that may add variety to their workout.

As you will see, yoga is a deeply philosophical art, although it can also be a healthy physical activity. We encourage you to try the exercises presented in this book. Follow the safety guidelines, and you will share in the enjoyment so many people have found from the practice of yoga!

About This Book

Yoga Basics offers the classic yoga postures, along with traditional breathing exercises and meditations to help you explore and expand your potential.

To introduce you to this ancient wisdom, the first three chapters present a brief look at yoga's history, philosophy, and classic systems. Practical information in Part II gets you started. The fundamental elements of yoga are explained next, in Part III: postures, breathing, and meditation. In Part IV you will find routines that will help you put the elements together into practice. Finally, Part V offers guidance for personalizing your practice of yoga.

part 1
introduction

THE PRACTICE OF YOGA is rooted in wisdom from the past. We draw our inspiration from ancient texts that laid the foundations. In the next three chapters, the history and philosophy of yoga are presented, with a look at the great works by creative thinkers from past centuries who have helped to shape yoga's destiny. Finally, the different forms of yoga, each with its own philosophical emphasis and practices, are discussed. Hatha yoga, combined with *raja* yoga and several of the other forms, is the emphasis of this book.

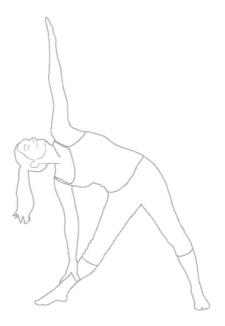

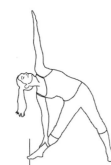

chapter 1
the history of yoga

Our actions still pursue us from afar,
And what we have been makes us what we are.
—*Radhakrishnan*

NDIA IS THE BIRTHPLACE of yoga. For thousands of years the Hindu people practiced and developed yoga, but unfortunately, much of yoga's historical beginnings in India have been lost in the passage of time.

Early gurus, teachers of yoga, taught students directly, rather than communicating their techniques through writing. Their students practiced yoga and developed many of the variations of postures, breathing, and meditation that we know today. Although the transmission of yoga was traditionally from teacher to student, there are a few main texts that have passed along the philosophy and practice of yoga.

One of India's great legacies to the world has been its philosophy, passed along through the ages by way of its profound Hindu texts, the *Vedas*. These spiritually oriented works influenced the early development of yoga.

The Texts

The *Vedas*

As many of the great philosophies can trace their root ideas back to lost ancient texts, so can yoga. Yoga's root themes were first vaguely expressed in the four ancient Hindu texts called the *Vedas: Rig, Yajur, Sama,* and *Atharva.* The *Vedas* are the earliest surviving writings of Indian thought, believed to be composed between 5000 and 2000 B.C. *Rig-Veda,* the best known, expresses spiritual knowledge in 1,028 lyrical hymns. Important yoga themes such as

> The *Upanishads* form the ending section of the *Vedas*, and so they present a culmination of the cultural teachings presented in the *Vedas*. They are also the foundation for future teachings of the later Indian philosophies. Their poetic style and deep underlying principles continue to inspire people today.

sacrifice, discipline, and praise for virtue and beauty are found in this work, but yoga techniques or methods are not clearly described.

The *Upanishads*

Yoga was more explicitly referred to later, in the *Upanishads*, written between 800 and 600 B.C. The title *Upanishads* comes from three sanskrit root words, *upa*, *ni* and *sad*, which collectively may be translated as "sitting down near," with the meaning of "receiving inner teachings." The philosophical meanings of the *Upanishads* are subject to varying interpretations, however. The concepts and doctrines first expressed in the *Upanishads* are echoed in all of the systems of Hindu philosophy that followed. The *Upanishads* instruct the seeker after truth to be moral and pure of heart, in order to perceive truth clearly. In the *Chandogya Upanishad*, a father teaches his son about truth by explaining that there is an inner essence in all things, which is their true nature, even though it is not evident through observation. The dialogues in the *Upanishads* encourage the seeker of this true nature to control the mind, and to control emotion. Then, just as a bright mirror reflects its surroundings, the mind will reflect reality. These ideas are the beginnings that led to yoga methods and techniques. A few *Upanishads* mention yoga in a primitive form. For example, the *Yoga Tattva Upanishad* specifically refers to aspects of yoga such as posture, breathing exercise, and mental training.

The *Mahabharata*

Although these texts are important, the most well known, early systematic description of yoga is found in the *Bhagavad-Gita*, which is a part of a larger Indian epic, the *Mahabharata*. Although its exact date is unknown, the *Bhagavad-Gita* was composed later than the *Upanishads*, between the fifth and second centuries B.C. Written as a dialogue between a warrior, Arjuna, and his charioteer, Krishna, this work lays out yoga philosophy in detail. Krishna's teachings define and explain the different branches of yoga, and although the *Bhagavad-Gita* was about the problems facing a warrior, this work makes it clear that yoga relates to all aspects of life. It shows how people can use yoga discipline to mold the clay of their lives and circumstances, to become what they want to be. The importance of the *Bhagavad-Gita* will be discussed further in the next chapter.

Patanjali's *Yoga Sutras*

Patanjali is recognized as the first to formally gather the practices of yoga into an ordered, consistent system. In his famous *Yoga Sutras*, compiled around A.D. 200, Patanjali explained that yoga is not just for physical well-being, but is also a philosophy for life. His concepts and general descriptions, originally of raja yoga, are now part of all yoga systems, in one form or another. His map of the eight stages, or limbs, of yoga set a pattern that all yoga systems use. Yoga's development follows a progression whose clear path can lead the practitioner from lower functioning to the mountain peak of enlightenment, through healthy and wholesome practices.

After the spread of Patanjali's *Yoga Sutras*, the teaching of yoga continued through direct transmission, from guru to student and down a line of succession. We will continue our discussion of the *Yoga Sutras* in the next chapter.

The word sutra translates as "thread" and is used to describe a work that connects ideas together into a meaningful whole.

The *Hatha Yoga Pradipika*

The first important written work to depict the postures used in hatha yoga is known as the *Hatha Yoga Pradipika*. This book not only described the practices, also included drawings of postures, but remained obscure and at first it was not translated. Other texts followed, all still in Indian languages.

Yoga Opens Its Doors

Many great yogis taught that truth and wisdom may be found in many philosophies and religions. *Yogi* is the word used to describe a committed practitioner of yoga. Because yoga is a philosophy of union, it is easily adaptable to other belief systems. As a result, various forms of spirituality have been combined with yoga as a means of gaining higher consciousness. This natural process developed gradually, making it impossible to determine exact dates.

Due to this adaptability, several kinds of Hindu yoga developed in India, such as Sankhya yoga, a combination of yoga with Sankhya philosophy. Certain sects of Buddhism also merged with yoga, for example the Yogacara School and Tibetan Buddhism. The Orient, Middle East, and Indonesia all received yoga and integrated it with their current practices. Even Christianity practices rituals that can be yogic in character, such as the meditation on the Stations of the Cross. As a result, the teaching of yoga continued to spread to more and more people, some of whom helped to facilitate the growth of yoga in a larger way.

Vivekananda Introduces Yoga to the West

In the late 1800s, some of the great Hindu yoga teachers began to open the doors of their ashrams to seekers from all over the world.

Vivekananda was the most significant early inspirational spokesman to bring yoga to the West. He opened the groundbreaking World Congress of Religions, held in Chicago in 1893. This meeting was the first time that religions such as Hinduism and Zen Buddhism were formally introduced to the West.

An ashram is a yoga sanctuary, and often the residence of a guru. During the late 1800s, ashrams became places of learning for students of yoga and Hinduism.

Vivekananda spoke passionately of tolerance and acceptance of all religions. He encouraged people to embrace an experience of universal oneness, linking all nations, religions, and people together with love and compassion. His philosophy embraced karma, bhakti, raja, and jnana yoga, as applications of yoga for different types of people with various lifestyles—he believed, for example, that working people would be inspired by karma yoga, while philosophically inclined intellectuals would prefer jnana yoga. He wrote a number of books and lectured widely, thoughtfully raising questions that are relevant to all humanity. Vivekananda devoted his life to guiding people toward what he believed was a higher truth concerning the inner true nature of humanity:

Krishnamurti's teachings continue to live on today through the Krishnamurti Foundation of America. Their mission is to preserve and disseminate the teachings of their founder, J. Krishnamurti. They do so through books, videos, lectures, and workshops. They are headquartered in Ojai, California.

"I shall not cease to work. I shall inspire men everywhere, until the world shall know that it is one with God." (Nikhilananda 1953, p. 179) Vivekananda was true to his word, and he spent his entire life spreading this message.

J. Krishnamurti Inspires the World's Youth

J. Krishnamurti was a jnana yogi who spoke on college campuses and engaged seekers of wisdom in dialogues throughout his long life, until his death in 1986. He masterfully showed his questioners how their own patterns of thinking created illusory obstacles to enlightened experience and living. He pointed out a way to follow that involved sensitivity and awareness, rather than techniques or methods of meditation. He believed that questioning deeply leads the questioner beyond thought into greater wisdom. Presenting his dialogues all over the world, Krishnamurti attempted to awaken people's minds to functioning on a deeper level, a level of unity. This statement captures his views:

> Such a mind is not a result, is not an end product of a practice, of meditation, of control. It comes into being from no form of discipline or compulsion or sublimation, without any effort of the "me", of thought; it comes into being when I understand the whole process of thinking—when I can see a fact without any distraction. In that state of tranquility of a mind that is really still there is love. And it is love alone that can solve all our human problems.
>
> (Krishnamurti 1968, p. 114)

Krishnamurti believed that when you think things through to their depth, you discover answers to life's questions.

Sri Aurobindo

Sri Aurobindo was an Indian who was raised and educated in England. His passion for India brought him back to his mother country, where he involved himself at first in political activity for Indian nationalism. But his nationalism soon became a spiritual quest instead, and his later years were devoted to conceiving, developing, and teaching a deeply philosophical integrated system of yoga. He believed in an evolutionary process leading to a pure consciousness-force—a super mind. Life, matter, and mind are all subordinate to super mind. "There is a double movement at work in Reality, declares Sri Aurobindo—a descent and an ascent." (Chaudhuri and Spiegelberg 1960, 300–301)

Aurobindo inspired his followers to do more and be more than they thought possible. He left a legacy through his many students and numerous books on philosophy and yoga. A modern example is spiritual teacher Sri Chinmoy and his own students, who continue to challenge and break limits of strength and endurance. Their feats are recorded in the *Guinness Book of World Records*. Some of the most famous feats are lifting 7,000 pounds, writing 1,300 books, painting thousands of paintings in a twenty-four-hour period, and learning to play hundreds of musical instruments.

Self-Realization Fellowship

Another early teacher of philosophical yoga was Paramahansa Yogananda, who came to Boston and founded the Self-Realization Fellowship in 1920. His system emphasized the religious application of yoga known as Kriya yoga. Today the fellowship has its headquarters in Los Angeles, California. The founder of Bikram yoga, Bikram Choudhury, was originally a student of Yogananda's brother, Bishnu Ghosh. As a religious practice, Kriya yoga emphasizes meditation.

Hatha Yoga Grand Masters

Several masters of yoga philosophy and practice were the cornerstones of modern Hatha yoga. They founded organizations that continue to spread their teachings today.

Krishnamacharya

Krishnamacharya was a great Hindu yoga master who taught and lived in India to the age of 101. He instructed at the palace of the Maharaja of Mysore. His students passed down their own lineages of yoga, which continue to have a strong influence on contemporary yoga teaching and philosophy. He was a shining example that showed how yoga can keep people healthy and youthful through their entire life. Many photographs of him in his late seventies and

> Krishnamacharya was a master teacher. The founder of several great systems of yoga (Iyengar and Ashtanga) were his students. His son continues to teach today.

eighties show him trim and fit, performing some of yoga's most challenging poses with grace, flexibility, and strength.

Krishnamacharya's son, Desikachar, continues to teach his father's system as taught to him. He includes postures, breathing, exercises, meditation methods, and philosophy of mind and conduct.

Krishnamacharya's younger brother-in-law, B.K.S. Iyengar, evolved a system of his own, which is widely taught, with a large number of postures and stretches. Although his system is firmly rooted in Krishnamacharya's, he was sent away to teach early in his career, and so developed his system using his own body to research his methods. He introduced the use of props such as blocks and straps to help students become more flexible and move more easily into the poses. Showing how yoga can be done at any age, Iyengar recently taught a large seminar with students from forty countries. He was eighty-two years old.

Another student of Krishnamacharya, Pattabhi Jois, founded the Ashtanga system of yoga, popular with young, active students. According to Ashtanga's history, Krishnamacharya and Jois discovered an ancient manuscript in a library, which Jois used along with Krishnamacharya's teachings to develop this system.

Indra Devi, a Russian student of Krishnamacharya, was the first woman yoga teacher in America. She came to California and taught many Hollywood celebrities, including Gloria Swanson, who posed for Devi's book on yoga, *Yoga for Americans*, in 1959.

Swami Sivananda

Swami Sivananda was an idealistic Hindu medical doctor who found himself drawn to yoga and ultimately chose yoga as his life's work. Many of his students came from Europe and America. He founded the Divine Life Society and developed an important system of yoga, Sivananda yoga, which is widely taught today. His prescription for a spiritual life was: "Serve, Love, Give, Purify, Meditate, Realize." (Lidell and Narayani 1983, p. 20) Sivananda's students included Satchidananda, who opened the famous Woodstock festival. His inspirational words were said to set the calm, spiritual tone for the memorable event: "The whole world is watching you. The entire world is going to know what American youth can do for humanity. America is helping everybody in the material field, but the time has come for America to help the whole world with spirituality also." (Satchidananda from www.integralyogaofnewyork.org)

Satchidananda founded the Integral Yoga Institute, and created a system that combines yoga with the Western philosophy of pragmatism to encourage higher functioning in body, mind, and spirit. Lilias Folan, a former well-known television yoga teacher, was part of this lineage as well.

Many other yoga teachers have come to America and Europe, too numerous to mention here, contributing their skill and wisdom to the world for the betterment of humanity.

Sivananda was an idealistic teacher who founded a large organization, the Divine Life Society. He taught widely and his students spread his teachings worldwide. Sivananda's approach emphasizes positive functioning of the body, mind, and spirit. He believed in harmony with all religions as sharing in spirituality.

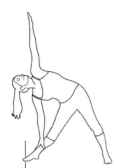

the philosophy
of yoga

*It is good to know that the ancient thinkers required
us to realize the possibilities of the soul in solitude and silence
and transform the flashing and fading moments of vision into
a steady light which could illuminate the long years of life.*
—*Radhakrishnan*

MORE THAN A PHILOSOPHY, yoga is a way of life. Yogic philosophy is optimistic; it teaches that with concentration, discipline, and proper technique, people can change their life patterns and destiny. Yoga allows you to transcend the limitations of an individual existence and unite with the greater universe. You can accomplish this through breathing, postures, and meditation practiced in the light of the philosophy of yoga. Although yoga falls under the larger umbrella of Hinduism, its philosophy has been expressed most clearly in two works, the *Bhagavad-Gita* and the *Yoga Sutras*.

The *Bhagavad-Gita*

The *Bhagavad-Gita* was one of the earliest statements of yoga philosophy. Written as a dialogue between Arjuna, a soldier from the warrior class, and Krishna, his charioteer, this epic spells out many of the basic concepts of yoga philosophy. Arjuna finds himself confronted with the uncomfortable task of fighting against relatives and friends for principles he believes in. He wishes he did not have to fight and considers avoiding his duty. Then he discusses the situation with Krishna. The charioteer explains courageous and positive ways to think and act in the situation Arjuna faces. Krishna's words reassure Arjuna and permit him to fully focus on his task. The dialogue gives him the courage and clear conscience to do what he must, wholeheartedly.

Through his teachings to Arjuna, Krishna defines and explains the branches of yoga. Since the word "yoga" is typically interpreted to mean yoking or uniting, the use of the metaphor of a charioteer is fitting: A charioteer yokes and controls the action of the chariot, just as yoga helps to unite the individual with the universal.

According to the *Bhagavad-Gita*, yoga is a method for uniting with, and being identified with, the spiritual universe. It teaches that you are real (physically existent) but that you also exist beyond the physical; you are not only your body. If you change in your body, for better or worse, you are still you, still the same person. There is something more within you, something eternal, transcending the body and its changes. To help people understand this idea, Satchidananda, renowned founder of the Integral Yoga Institute, stated that when he died, the teachings would not die with him. The principles transcend the physical person who expresses them. You can discover the source as well. Conscious and unconscious work together, united by concentration, to accomplish great things.

Yoga unites our individual existence with the larger universe. Many of the great yoga teachers point us to a larger perspective as the source for deeper wisdom.

The *Bhagavad-Gita* states that we all have a duty to work, but not as slaves. Work can be the source of freedom. People will be free when they do good for the sake of doing good. Krishna explains that action should not arise out of fear of consequences or out of selfish motives. In this way, Krishna encourages Arjuna to be unattached to the fruits of action. "Therefore, always perform the work that has to be done without attachment, for man attains the Supreme by performing work without attachment." (Deutsch 1968, p. 49) Vivekananda expressed this idea idealistically when he told people to work with love and self-sacrifice, not just for return.

Central to the philosophy in the *Bhagavad-Gita* is that roles or actions, when performed morally, correctly, and wholeheartedly, can be liberating and need not be feared or shunned. Morality is necessary. Yoga philosophy involves will, focus, and conscious control of the mind, in order to transcend the body. The body and mind can be trained deliberately to bring about enlightenment. Mind and body are one: do not dissociate them. "The highest Self of him who has conquered the self and is peaceful remains ever concentrated in heat and cold, pleasure and pain, in honor and dishonor." (Deutsch 1968, p. 66)

All paths are one path, leading to the higher purpose. Your experiences are teachers, your path to walk on to find your higher self. The steps of yoga lead to completion, although each has its own set of practices. When combined, they result in enlightenment, known as *samadhi*, union, Oneness.

The *Yoga Sutras* and the Eight Limbs of Yoga

Patanjali claimed that he was not creating something new in his sutras, but was gathering together ancient wisdom that had been taught for centuries, teacher to student.

More than any other text on yoga, the *Yoga Sutras* show that yoga is a philosophy of action for living, not just a set of exercises. Written by Patanjali, the *Yoga Sutras* describe, in very brief, terse language, how the process of yoga comes about, what it is, and its benefits for practitioners. The legendary story of Patanjali's birth portends his important writings. It relates that a newborn serpent fell into the cupped hands of his mother, while she was offering water in worship of the sun. She named her son Patanjali from *pata*, meaning "falling serpent" and *anjah*, meaning the cupped gesture of her hands, or "worshipping." The serpent took on human form in order to write for the benefit of mankind. Patanjali stated that he was not the originator. He was merely the gatherer of ancient wisdom.

Patanjali included within his sutras a general code of conduct to help guide practitioners. Progress is based on the Eight Limbs of Yoga, a step-by-step process. Like rungs on a ladder, each step requires the step earlier, and the earlier steps form the basis for the later steps. For example, before meditation is possible, *yamas* (what you should abstain from doing) and *niyamas* (what you should do) must be sincerely lived, not just thought about. The flow of yoga is continuous, giving direction and guidance to the life force.

Ahimsa, the yama of nonharming, not only refers to not hurting other people, but also implies not hurting yourself. Yoga practice is healthy and life-promoting. People are encouraged to make positive lifestyle choices and avoid anything that is harmful, as expressed in the value of ahimsa.

The First Two Limbs: the Yamas and Niyamas

There are five yamas and five niyamas. These guides to conduct and practice are basic to an ethically committed yogic life. The great religious leader and humanitarian Mahatma Gandhi incorporated the yamas and niyamas into his personal conduct. His theory of action and nonviolence was drawn from the ancient wisdom of the yamas: "I have nothing new to teach the world. Truth and nonviolence are as old as the hills." (Kripalani 1960, p. 1)

The Yamas

Ahimsa, the first yama, means "nonharming" and is interpreted as nonviolence. In a general sense, this means that you should try not to do any harm to anyone at any time, including yourself: nonviolence in thought, word, and action. Vegetarianism is a good example of ahisma, because yogis don't want to harm any creature.

Ahimsa can be the yoga practitioner's basis for kindness toward others. Along with ahimsa, according to Iyengar, goes freedom from fear, and freedom from anger. Leading a pure life brings about freedom from fear. The spirit within transcends old age, sickness, decay, and even death. Yoga practitioners dedicate personal existence to higher purposes. They give up anger toward others. And though they may have faults, they should be gentle toward others. No one should want to harm others with anger or hostility. So the practitioner cultivates benevolent, nonagressive responses.

Satya, the second yama, means not lying. Being false will prevent you from staying on the true yoga path. Never lying leads to being truthful—sincere in thought, word, and deed. Real, authentic communication with others results in thoughtfulness.

Satya is fundamental in yoga. Truth means more than not lying. Truthfulness is part of the nature of greater wisdom. Yoga doctrines aim toward higher truths, so a deep commitment to truth helps the practitioner stay on track to greater wisdom. Deception, however slight, leads away from truth, and thus yoga philosophy values truth highly.

For example, in cabinetmaking and house building, truth is a central issue.

When a beam is level, it is called true. When a unit is correctly angled with a right angle, or a forty-five-degree miter, it is also called true. We commonly speak of being true to form, or of telling the truth. In law we swear to tell the truth, as the basis of justice. All of these examples show how significant truth is, even in our own system of values. Valuing truth is basic to yoga as well.

The third yama, *brahmacharya*, is restraint and control, moderation of enjoyment through the senses. Gandhi said, "A certain degree of physical harmony and comfort is necessary, but above that level, it becomes a hindrance instead of a help." (Kripalani 1960, p. 140) Some interpret brahmacharya to mean refinement and purification of intimate relationships so that personal involvement matters. Relationships should be sincere and moderate, honorably true to the partner, not promiscuous and liberal. Some practitioners interpret it as complete abstinence from sensual pleasure, while others believe that it only means one should not be promiscuous. This yama naturally leads to being selective and moderate in sexual relationships. But brahmacharya can refer to a much broader category than just intimate relationships. Brahmacharya is an attitude of purity of mind and heart that can extend to all aspects of life. Thus, ethics and spirituality become integrated with everyday life.

> Simplicity is a value held by many philosophies of higher consciousness. When you have your heart set on deeper wisdom, material needs lose some of their allure and can take their rightful place as just one aspect of a happy life.

Asteya, the fourth yama, is non-stealing. You should resist the temptation to take anything that does not belong to you. The concept of this yama also can include nonpossession of someone else's thought, word, or action. The result is that, just as you do not take other people's goods, you also do not take on other people's negative ideas or opinions, or adopt their negative actions. You should free yourself by letting them go. This is asteya.

The fifth yama is *aparigraha*, or rejection of greed. Some view this as being nongrasping. This yama asks people to cultivate detachment and not be greedy for things they don't really need. Aparigraha helps to moderate your desire for possessions and acquisitions. Observance of this yama leads to generosity in thought, work, and action. And cultivating moderation leads to a simpler life, with fewer needs. This yama frees practitioners from lower concerns and turns them to higher purposes.

The Niyamas

The niyamas are a code of conduct people should adopt. *Shaucha* is the first niyama and refers to purity, cleanliness, and neatness of body, mind, and spirit. This includes special cleansing methods and purification. Outwardly, the house should be clean and neat, the person well-groomed and clean. Food should be pure, toxin-free, natural, and healthy. The place of yoga practice should be pure as well. Inner cleanliness also involves clarity of mind brought about by the practice of asanas, pranayama, and meditation. Thus, meditation and breathing methods help one to find the path, but shaucha orients, showing the direction.

To evolve, self-awareness must be cultivated. When it is practiced deliberately and focused on, self-awareness grows. *Samtosha*, the second niyama, is the development of self-awareness and balanced nonattachment. The observance of this niyama results in contentment toward yourself, your belongings, and your environment. Learn how to appreciate what you have; learn to accept what happens in your life, and learn from it.

The third niyama, *tapas*, is physical austerity, which leads to fitness of body and mind. Tapas involves practicing asanas, pranayama, and meditation as you make an effort to change and improve. Discipline is part of this. Paying attention to your eating habits, posture, and breathing patterns helps to keep you fit and healthy.

Hatha yoga is intimately integrated with tapas. It is the basis of a healthy, fitness-oriented lifestyle, which promotes long life and spirituality. Mind, body, and spirit work together with implementation of tapas.

Svadhyaya, the fourth niyama, refers to inquiry or examination. This niyama encourages study, memorization, and contemplation of great literature, along with self-study and reflection. In order to practice this niyama, you can read the great literature of Hinduism such as the *Mahabharata* or the *Vedas*, or study biographies of yoga masters. Whatever you choose to read, it is important not to neglect the development of your intellect. So if you are from the Judeo-Christian tradition, you may want to read the Bible, while Buddhists may want to read the great sutras. Self-study and learning keep you properly on the path.

The fifth niyama, *isvara pranidhana*, is dedication to a higher power, whether this means surrender to God's will, yielding to nature's design, or following another path. This niyama encourages you to make your best spiritual efforts wholeheartedly while "letting be"—surrendering to the spontaneous unfolding of the present moment, being one with the here and now, and staying in the here and now without concern for the future or past. Yoga teacher Satchidananda told people to believe in Now. Be deeply one with your life as it is, and have faith in it. Believe in believing itself, not just in a particular belief. Belief and faith can lead to wisdom and higher truth, through this niyama.

Asana and Pranayama

The third limb of yoga is asana, the practice of postures that unite the mind and body. Pranayama is the fourth limb of yoga, directing and integrating the breath and life force. Pranayama is the practice of varying breathing patterns while contemplating internal or external objects. A large part of this book is devoted to asanas, pranayama, and the next limb of yoga, meditation.

Pratyahara, Dharana, Dhyana, and Samadhi

The next three limbs involve mental skills developed through meditation and disciplined practice. *Pratyahara*, the fifth, is pulling back the senses from focusing on the external world and directing them toward the inner self, the soul. Pratyahara is followed by *dharana*, one-pointed, focused concentration on the object of attention. Fully immersed, the mind goes to the state of *dhyana*, the seventh limb. Dhyana is contemplation or meditation, the flow of consciousness that leads to the eighth limb, the experience of *samadhi*, oneness, enlightenment, dissolving into the sea of the universe. In raja yoga, great abilities and powers are believed to come from this process.

Most modern schools of yoga follow this patterned sequence of the eight limbs. The limbs of yoga lead to the ultimate goal of higher consciousness, transcendent awareness in which we realize our true self, at one with the universal Self.

For the yoga practitioner, everyday life continually offers opportunities, beginning with observing the restraints of the yamas and niyamas, through practicing asana postures and pranayama breathing, to withdrawal, concentration, contemplation, and enlightenment.

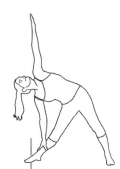

chapter 3
the different
forms of yoga

Practice is basically the correct effort required to move
toward, reach, and maintain the state of Yoga.
—*Patanjali*

THE DISCIPLINES OF YOGA were originally thought of as separate paths, but later many of them were combined. Each form of yoga helps to concentrate attention toward a particular point of focus, bringing about self-discipline and leading to a state of samadhi, enlightenment. Combined, the different forms of yoga could have a more comprehensive effect by developing mind, body, and spirit together. Vivekananda, with his visionary optimism, hoped to influence the unification of the forms of yoga. His lifelong commitment was to seeing all religions come together. He said, "All religions and all spiritual disciplines lead to one and the same goal." (Nikhilananda 1953, p. 503)

Some of the most commonly practiced forms of yoga are hatha yoga, raja yoga, jnana yoga, karma yoga, bhakti yoga, mantra yoga, yantra yoga, and tantra yoga.

Hatha yoga is the form of yoga best known to the West and now includes other forms in its practice. Hatha yoga is the yoga of health, with many types of postures, breathing methods, and meditation to enhance vitality and well-being. Hatha yoga is a central focus of this book.

Raja Yoga

Raja yoga is known as royal yoga, specializing in the development of the mind, consciousness, and character. Based on Patanjali's eight limbs, raja yoga helps

> Some separate yoga disciplines have unified with each other, so that each is rarely taught in complete isolation from the other. The distinctions of each discipline remain, but they are complementary.

people develop themselves to their highest potential for enlightened wisdom. The practice of raja yoga includes asanas, pranayama, and meditation, but it tends to emphasize moving through higher and higher levels of meditation.

Rather than seeking wisdom through rational thought, raja yoga practitioners use meditative methods and techniques of attention, concentration, and contemplation. These meditative methods are then used for discipline, control, and direction of the mind.

Raja yoga includes many methods of meditation and concentration that lead to higher consciousness. For example, in one technique practitioners are told to imagine a lotus on top of their head, several inches up, with virtue as its center and knowledge as its stalk. Thus the focus of concentration is symbolic, to help lead the meditator into higher consciousness.

Enlightenment is also fostered through deliberate practice. Another meditation is to imagine a space in your heart and visualize a flame burning. Then imagine that the flame is your own soul and that inside that flame is another light, the higher soul. This meditation encourages unity between our own individuality and the greater universe.

In modern practice, raja yoga is often combined with hatha yoga, as in this book. These kinds of raja yoga meditations, when combined with postures and breathing, can help people to gain mental skills and find Nirvana.

Jnana Yoga

Jnana yoga is the yoga of wisdom. It is a philosophical investigation of life, the search for true wisdom. Followers of this path contemplate life, using conceptual, rational thought to turn the mind toward higher consciousness. They look at the larger perspective and ask important questions: Why do we need religion? What is the nature of humanity? What is true wisdom? What is death? How can we understand ourselves?

Practitioners of jnana yoga believe that if you reason back to the roots, you will discover truth. Most of the time, however, people are deceived. "Because we talk in vain, and because we are satisfied with the things of the senses, and

> Meditation is the method that allows us to experience our Oneness with the greater universe. Through careful practice of focused attention, people learn how to let go of the boundaries of their individual ego and sense their connection with the world.

because we are running after desires, therefore, we cover the Reality, as it were, with a mist." (Nikhilananda 1953, p. 219) This world of illusion is called *maya*, and jnana yoga tries to clear away the mist of maya to find the truth about reality.

A renowned exemplar of jnana yoga is J. Krishnamurti. He believed that it is important to discover truths about ourselves and our world by inner exploration: A transformation of the world is brought about by a transformation of oneself. This is one of the basic beliefs in jnana yoga. Jnana yoga can inspire us to reach beyond our everyday existence, to seek deeper and make discoveries. "As we understand the near, we shall find the distance between the near and the far is not. There is no distance—the beginning and the end are one." (Krishnamurti 1968, p. 176)

Karma Yoga

Karma yoga is the practice of applying yoga to everyday life, for achieving enlightened living and higher goals. The word "karma" comes from the Sanskrit word *kri*, meaning "to do," and in karma yoga, it refers to working. Karma yoga is very useful for those who seek enlightenment while also wishing to be in the everyday world, raising a family or developing a career or occupation. Karma yoga teaches practitioners to maintain their focus in the midst of life. "The calmer we are and the less disturbed our nerves, the more shall we love and the better will our work be." (Nikhilananda 1953, p. 486)

Every person has his or her own unique individual nature with certain talents and capacities. Karma yoga calls upon us to fulfill our potential, to do something that matters. In fact, these yogis believe that it is our duty to be the best that we can. This idea calls upon us to struggle to live up to our own highest ideals. We should strive to live lives that are as close to our ideals as possible.

Every person should set goals and then try to accomplish them. This theme is seen in yoga practice generally. We are urged to set goals for our yoga practice and then make every effort to follow through with them (see chapter 19).

The *Bhagavad-Gita* clearly described the fundamental doctrine of karma yoga: to develop nonattachment. Work that is performed for selfish gain will not lead you to higher consciousness. But work that is performed with nonattachment, with your self detached from the fruits of your labor, will bring true happiness.

Students of karma yoga analyze their thoughts and their actions to learn about different qualities of thinking and behaving, to help them channel their actions correctly. They train to be able to accept what is and not be worried or swayed by it. Thought and action are the focus for meditation.

Yogis who practice karma yoga engage selflessly in their work, their relationships, and their lives. They engage in everything they do as fully and awarely as possible, but they gain no personal satisfaction from a job well done. The higher purpose is more significant to them. So they don't need to look outside themselves for approval, and are not easily pushed off-course by difficulties. They have developed the inner strength and determination to stay focused and committed to whatever they do, for the sake of others, and for the sake of love. Personal motives are not the source of karma yoga actions, in work or relationships.

> Karma yoga has relevance to people today, as it helps us to develop higher consciousness through work. Work can be a meaningful and fulfilling part of life if we approach it in the right way.

Thus, karma yoga urges people to do the very best they can in their social roles. What really matters is the fact of doing well for its own sake, not for gain. People should use commitment to work, family life, and social life as an opportunity to develop fully.

Bhakti Yoga

Bhakti yoga is the yoga of devotion and selfless love. Bhakti yoga includes methods and ideas for finding enlightenment through compassion and charitable actions. "When a man gets it, he loves all, hates none; he becomes satisfied for ever." (Nikhilananda 1953, p. 405) According to Vivekananda, bhakti yoga can be a very accessible and natural way to reach Nirvana. He

Tantra techniques are ancient and found in many different cultures, so no one knows its exact origin. The Sanskrit word *tantra* implies "continuation," and "weaving together," but there is no single definition. Tantra includes many sets of techniques, usually action-oriented, to weave together body and mind.

cautions that people should not interpret the loving devotion of bhakti yoga too narrowly. For example, people should not limit their own ideas about what or whom to love. Bhakti yoga is universal love.

Bhakti yoga is divided into two stages. The first is *gauni*, the preparatory stage, and the second is *para*, the supreme stage. Bhakti yogis perform a succession of meditations, directed toward a religious realization. This practice may begin with ordinary worship, but eventually it leads to a deep spiritual realization.

Bhakti yogis immerse themselves in dedicated actions by doing work in charitable organizations for the benefit of a group or for the greater benefit of humanity. Bhakti yoga helps practitioners to find the higher universal Self through letting go of the small individual self and its self-centered concerns. Krishna Consciousness is a modern Bhakti yoga organization.

Tantra Yoga

Tantra yoga is an action-oriented yoga most notably used in Tibetan Buddhism. This form of yoga seeks enlightenment through sensual and emotional experiences, which may include a relationship with a partner. It is the goal of tantra yoga to expand awareness in all states of consciousness.

Tantra yoga assumes that desires are the primary motivators in life. Rather than asking people to renounce desires, tantric yogis view desire as natural. Therefore, to master ourselves, we need to develop a shift in consciousness. Tantric yogis teach people how to use their senses, desires, and all aspects of life as symbols of higher consciousness. Everything in life can become an opportunity to exercise yoga discipline for higher consciousness.

The six *chakras* are psychic centers in the body. Desires are directly related to the six psychic centers. Meditation and breathing techniques can teach people how to master their desires and direct their energy to create a bridge connecting mind, body, and spirit.

Tantric yoga meditation develops one-pointed awareness to free consciousness from its limitations. Meditation techniques include many kinds of concentration exercises designed to help you learn to narrow the focus of concentration and sustain this one-pointed direction.

Tantra yoga also enlists all the senses in the search for enlightenment. Thus, the tactile, visual, and auditory senses are developed and used in creative techniques and meditations. Tantra yoga includes practices for training partners to enhance sexual relationships. These sexual techniques also teach practitioners to merge with their partner and, thereby, with the greater universe. Intimate relationships can then become a way of attuning to the symbolic level of experience.

Mandalas and yantras are visual tools to help people center themselves in the symbolic, through the sense of sight. Mandalas are circular pictures with symbolic shapes and figures that represent the universe. Yantras are a type of mandala with geometric shapes that are used as a focal point for meditation. Both yantras and mandalas are used as objects of meditation.

Mantras are an auditory tool of tantra yoga. One of the most famous mantras, om, is "the symbolic word for the infinite, the perfect, the eternal." (Simpkins 2001, p. 49)

Mantra Yoga

Mantras are also basic to their own yoga, called mantra yoga. Mantra yoga is the yoga of sound. It uses repetitions of sounds, syllables, and phrases to bring about changes in consciousness. A well-known example of this is Transcendental Meditation, also known as T.M., as taught by Maharishi Mahesh Yogi. T.M. trains students to meditate with their own personal, specially chosen mantra. By focusing attention fully on the sound of their mantra, people can bring about a personal evolution toward enlightened consciousness.

All of these many paths lead to the same goal. Yoga has many varieties of practices, which in classical form were distinct and separate. In modern practice, they tend to be integrated, sharing a common root in their sincere devotion to the enhancement of human potential. Today, yoga schools offer alternatives within their curriculum. Therefore, jnana yoga, the yoga of wisdom, may be practiced in combination with karma yoga, the yoga of working people, for wiser, more enlightened living. Mantra yoga, the yoga of sound, may be used with hatha yoga to intensify practice and development.

part 2
getting started

A YOGA PRACTICE that starts out thoughtfully and with awareness will bring more enjoyment and greater benefit, and for this reason part 2 guides you in getting started in yoga. Chapter four describes the many schools available, to help you choose the best school for you. Some of the aids used in yoga practice are described in chapter 6. Safety should always be considered, and chapter 7 explains how to practice yoga safely. The final chapter in this section, chapter 8, will prepare you for your first routine, with warmups and instruction on how to begin.

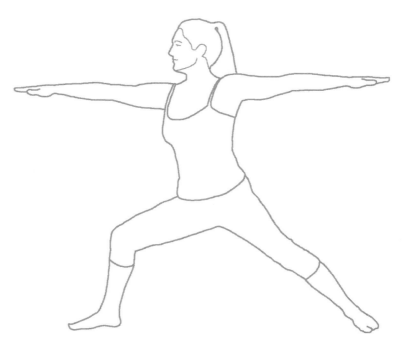

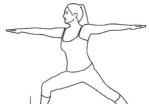

chapter 4
choosing the right
style of yoga for you

To succeed you must have tremendous perseverance, tremendous will.
"I will drink the ocean," says the persevering soul, "And at my will,
mountains will crumble." Have that sort of energy, that sort of will,
work hard, and you will reach the goal.
— *Vivekananda*

MODERN YOGA SCHOOLS often offer varieties of traditional yoga practices. Thus, although most yoga classes include similar postures, they vary the emphasis and teaching to match the philosophy of the style. All approaches can be good; which one you follow will depend on what you are looking for and on your individual needs.

The styles described here represent a sampling of some of the mainstream larger organizations in the West. These descriptions can help you sort out some of the choices that are available and give you guidelines for deciding what will fit your needs. You may find an excellent school that combines these traditions or differs from them slightly. Your ultimate choice should include your personal assessment of the situation and how well you feel that the approach fits you.

> There are many different styles of yoga, each with its own emphasis and orientation. Drawn from the same roots, they share in the basic principles of yoga. But the variations make room for all kinds of practitioners with different levels of interest and needs.

Ashtanga Vinyasa Yoga

If you are limber and want the challenge of an energetic workout, Ashtanga may be best for you. Ashtanga was created by one of Krishnamacharya's students, Pattabhi Jois. *Ashtanga* means eight-limbed, and *vinyasa* means breathing system. Sometimes known as power yoga, Ashtanga yoga concentrates on demanding physical practice to lead students to the upper levels of meditation. This form of yoga is 95 percent action and 5 percent philoso-

> **A**shtanga yoga is usually taught as a very intense and demanding form, appealing most frequently to people who are already somewhat fit or athletic.

phy. Thus, the philosophy is experienced through the activity of doing the asanas, pranayama, and meditation. Ashtanga yoga tends to be very active. There are, of course, gradations of the intensity, but the intent of the Ashtanga system is to push toward your limits in order to extend them. Ashtanga classes are usually divided into beginner, intermediate, and advanced so that you can progress at the pace you need. Each level of class has an appropriate routine, which you come to expect at every workout.

The class begins with dynamic breathing into movement, one posture flowing into the next with little pause. "Dynamic" in yoga refers to moving, so as practitioners move into and out of postures, they coordinate their breathing with the motions. Next come static poses that are held for a period of time. Breathing techniques are also coordinated with every pose. Breath is life according to Ashtanga yoga, so constant interweaving of breathing and movement helps weave them into one. The exercises also include several specialized pranayama locking techniques called *bandhas*, as well as meditation. Students learn how to lock their breath into certain areas such as the throat or the abdomen. These techniques help students to develop advanced levels of breath control.

The specialized pranayama techniques in Ashtanga help raise internal heat. Practitioners of Ashtanga believe that this heating process will nourish and purify the body systems. So you can expect to sweat in these workouts while developing extreme flexibility and vital energy. The guru's input is central in helping students to achieve high levels of skill.

Bikram Yoga

If you want a reliable, systematic approach to yoga that does not vary from the first day on and gives an overall workout, then Bikram yoga may be suited to you.

> **B**ikram yoga offers a stable workout, day after day, that always includes the same basic elements. By continuing to perfect the workout over time, practitioners gain skill and proficiency while also experiencing the spiritual benefits that yoga practice can bring.

Bikram Choudhury founded the Yoga College of India in Beverly Hills, California, in 1974. Bikram combined ancient yoga doctrines with scientific input from doctors at the Tokyo University Hospital to put together a modernized and standardized workout.

Bikram yoga is an intelligently designed series of twenty-six postures that works the body from the inside out. Each posture strengthens and stretches the muscles for the next posture. Breathing is coordinated with the postures, and there are also separate breathing exercises. Bikram yoga also trains the mind through meditation to improve self-control, determination, concentration, and patience.

Another feature of a Bikram workout is that the room is heated to approximately 90 degrees in order to relax muscles and to sweat out toxins. Even though a Bikram workout is intensive, the style is open to all ages and all levels. The instructor should help you pace yourself correctly as you get started.

Iyengar Yoga

If you want a complete lifestyle practice, with meditation, breathing, postures, and an overall holistic emphasis, Iyengar yoga may be your choice. This style draws upon a wide variety of postures and props to help you learn with ease. Because Iyengar yoga offers a slower-paced and individualized curriculum, it can be used for therapeutic purposes, to overcome injuries, and as a good starting place for beginners. But Iyengar yoga also takes advanced students deeply into the yoga experience. This style has a creative, flexible curriculum to keep the class fresh and new.

The Iyengar system uses props such as chairs, blocks, straps, pillows, and mats to make for a more gradual easing into the postures. The class teaches many creative uses of these props to help people achieve more than they thought possible.

Each class emphasizes different themes. For example, one class might be devoted to stretching the back, another to limbering the hips or strengthening the chest. With so many poses and ways to perform them, each area can be developed creatively.

Integral Yoga

Spiritually oriented students who also seek health may gravitate toward Integral yoga. Integral yoga is a synthesis of methods and philosophy to develop all sides of the spiritual seeker. It combines many forms of yoga, including hatha, raja, karma, bhakti, and jnana. It also incorporates the use of mantras through *japa* yoga, divine vibration. The goal of Integral yoga is to realize spiritual unity and live in harmony with yourself and the greater universe. This is achieved through the practice of five basic principles: relaxation, exercise, breathing, diet, and meditation. Thus, Integral yoga classes have a soothing atmosphere. Incense fills the slightly shaded room. Each class includes breathing exercises, postures, and meditation. Sound is also incorporated through mantras.

Yoga practice can bring a transformation of the inner person. Lifestyle becomes healthier and everyday life is more fulfilling. Integral yoga addresses itself to the whole person, helping to harmonize yoga practice into everyday living.

Class usually starts with the sun salutation and then goes through a series of postures. More advanced students perform cycles of each posture that carefully work the position even more deeply. Students begin holding positions very briefly and gradually learn to hold them for longer periods of time.

Integral yoga offers a good overall workout for people of all ages and at any level. It also gives guidance toward a well-rounded, healthier balance of mind, body, and spirit.

Kripalu Yoga

Those who are looking for a gentler approach to yoga may like Kripalu yoga. The Kripalu Center for Yoga and Health headquartered in Lenox, Massachusetts, is one of the largest yoga and holistic centers in the United States. The founder, Yogi Amrit Desai, named the style after his guru, Swami Kripalvananda.

This form of yoga has a reputation for being moderate in its approach. It offers a step-by-step introduction into yoga practice by starting with the basic asanas and building gradually from there. Kripalu yoga instructors believe that people will find deep and lasting benefits by easing themselves into the practice of yoga. The Kripalu Center also offers a Web site that gives encouragement and instructions for basic postures.

Asanas, pranayama, and meditation are practiced in the traditional way. But innovations are also integrated into practice at the Center. For example, partner massages and lectures on holistic health are also offered. Students can attend regularly scheduled classes. More intensive experiences that offer other styles to supplement Kripalu, such as Ashtanga, are also available through classes and overnight retreats. In this way the Kripalu Center presents a broad range of yoga approaches. Kripalu classes taught by certified Kripalu teachers are available in many locations around the world.

Kundalini Yoga

Students who are fascinated by some of the esoteric breathing techniques of yoga might like to try kundalini yoga. This is a modern approach that draws its name from the traditional kundalini practice of awakening the body's cosmic energy (see Chapter 12). This style teaches students to awaken their kundalini energy through breathing and meditation techniques. But some kundalini yoga schools also teach the traditional asanas, pranayama, and meditation along with chanting, bandhas (locking techniques), and mudras (symbolic hand positions). Kundalini yoga is a tantric method that helps people unify mind and body as they discover a higher state of consciousness.

Yoga has a mystical dimension and kundalini yoga addresses this side of yoga through its practice of kundalini energy meditations.

finding a yoga class

Breathe as you enter into each pose
Concentrate deeply, change flows
Leave the unchangeable past behind
Happiness begins now with an open mind
—*C. Alexander Simpkins*

YOU MAY WANT TO supplement your home workout by attending a regular class. When you begin exploring the different yoga schools in your area, you may be faced with a bewildering number of possibilities! Many different options are available, so you can probably find the class format that suits you best.

Which Class Is for You?

The different forms of yoga discussed in chapter 4 can serve as a general guideline. Many of these styles are available in their pure form. The Yoga College of India offers Bikram yoga. Iyengar yoga is another pure style that can

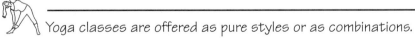

Yoga classes are offered as pure styles or as combinations.

be found in the West. Ashtanga is also available as a pure form of yoga. But you are likely to also find that many of the schools do not practice just one form alone. A large percent of them combine different forms of yoga. So you may see Ashtanga and Iyengar offered together at your local yoga center.

Every type of person can find a suitable yoga class. Modern yoga centers are offering classes that target unique needs for particular situations.

The combinations can be even more creative today. Yoga is being taught along with tai chi, Buddhism, Zen, Pilates, and hypnosis. Massage is also commonly included as an option. Some centers are oriented toward health and fitness. You will find yoga classes offered at fitness clubs as well as at some martial arts studios.

Classes vary in their environment as well. Some are spiritually oriented. They might burn incense and lower the lights to create a meditative atmosphere. A more fitness-oriented class will be done in a gym or health club aerobics room. You can expect to get different results depending upon whether the class is geared more to spirituality or physical fitness. But most schools provide a combination of these two qualities, since yoga always involves the mind and body working together. So yoga will give you a great workout while also developing your mental powers through meditation and breathing.

Another new development is yoga for various select populations. You can find yoga for golfers, healing yoga for people recovering from injuries, yoga for pregnant women, yoga for the elderly and the young. Yoga has also been incorporated into a "yogatherapy" for personal growth and stress management. These yoga classes combine body work with the mental calming and centering of meditation and breathing, to help people lower their discomfort and make healthier adjustments to the stresses of life. Athletes can get better performance by supplementing their training with yoga classes. Strength, flexibility, and concentration can be improved, all important components for many sports.

Despite all the variations, the actual postures performed tend to be universal. Almost all schools will do the asanas included in this book. Your home sessions will coordinate well with most classes.

You will get a good sense of the class and how it seems to fit your needs by observing a typical class, so you should consider personally visiting the yoga class you are considering. Most schools are very welcoming and will be happy to let you watch a class if you like.

Finding a Yoga Teacher

Traditionally in yoga, the relationship with a teacher was most important. The yoga teacher was a guru, a spiritual guide. Students became disciples of their guru, spending many years of study, not just practicing the postures, but also delving deeply into yoga literature and philosophy. The process led to a life-altering transformation in the student. Vivekananda established a number of qualifications for yoga teachers that might help you with your decision. Teachers should be knowledgeable in the spirit and literature of yoga. They should also be moral, with a strong character. Teachers should not be driven by selfish motives.

Today you will find a great variety of choices. Well-known gurus from the East have set up centers in certain locations around the country. If you are interested in making a deep commitment to a particular guru, you may be able to study with him or her directly at the central location. More commonly, people are looking for an enjoyable class to attend a few times per week. Most yoga teachers offer a class situation with many students practicing together. The depth of your relationship with the teacher can vary, depending upon your own needs. A teacher whom you trust will help bring out the best in you, or point the way for you to discover your own path. The person-to-person contact of a good instructor can help you to develop your potential.

A yoga instructor can be more than just a person who teaches yoga. Some yoga instructors are gurus, enlightened individuals who guide students toward spiritual awakening.

Find out about the background of your potential teacher. Some of the traditional styles offer a certification process with ethical codes and standards for their members. There are a number of large organizations that certify teachers from diverse styles as well, such as the Yoga Alliance, which registers yoga teachers who have met certain minimum standards. These credentials require a certain number of years of practice plus a set number of hours of training, and an agreement to abide by a code of ethics. And of course, for your personal development, you may need to take other qualities into account. How many years has the teacher been practicing yoga? How long has he or she taught?

Although yoga has not established a universal credentialing system, there is a widespread movement toward establishing a benchmark for ethics and conduct. The diverse teaching styles and methods all share a common root in the ethics of the yamas and niyamas. You can expect a commitment to ethical conduct from your yoga school.

When choosing a yoga class, carefully gather information, observe the class, and talk to the instructor. But don't ignore your intuitive sense of the situation. Yoga works on many levels, so allow yourself to be open to all the resources available from outside and within.

As you observe a class, consider the teacher's manner with the students. Does each student get appropriate attention? Does the teacher seem professionally involved and caring? How knowledgeable and skilled is this teacher? Try to imagine yourself as a student in the student-to-teacher relationship. Does it fit your needs?

Another important issue in yoga is how the teacher guides the students into correct position. Some teachers will strongly move students to correct their pose, while others are more gentle and cautious with their touch. A more vigorous and dynamic approach may be suitable for a flexible, athletic individual who wants to be pushed to peak performance. But this kind of teaching could cause discomfort, or perhaps even injury, to the person needing a more gradual building of skills. Be sensitive to your needs, and you will progress.

Yoga includes ethics in the yamas and niyamas, so teachers should be ethical in the way they conduct their classes. Look for a forthright disclosure of rates, times, and size of classes.

Before you begin, find out what you need to bring or purchase. Some schools will require that you bring your own mat. Some may ask you to buy equipment, while others may provide aids in the class for use.

Making Your Choice

Ramakrishna, the teacher of Vivekananda, told a story that conveys some good common-sense advice. A group of people wanted to learn about the quality of the mangos in an orchard. They counted the leaves, twigs, and branches of the mango trees. They examined the color, size, and weight of the fruit. Then they gathered together to discuss their findings. Meanwhile, another person entered the grove. He took a mango and began eating it. Ramakrishna asks, "Was this other person not wise?"

Don't ignore your personal reactions to the teacher and the class. Do you like the teacher? Does the class seem to fit your personality? Are you comfortable in this classroom setting? Your own intuitive sense of all these factors should be included as part of your decision.

Once you have decided on a class, give it a try before you make a longer commitment. Actually doing the class may be different from just watching. If you have chosen well, your experience will be enjoyable and enriching!

props and clothes

The young, the old, the extremely aged, even the sick and the infirm obtain perfection in Yoga by constant practice. Success will follow him who practices, not him who practices not. Success in Yoga is not obtained by the mere theoretical reading of sacred texts. Success is not obtained by wearing the dress of a yogi or a sannyasi (a recluse), nor by talking about it. Constant practice alone is the secret of success. Verily, there is no doubt of this. —Hatha Yoga Pradipika

THE MOST IMPORTANT requirement for success with yoga is your own willingness to do it. As the above quote says, success will only come with practice, and people have invented a number of aids to help you advance, to enhance safety, and to encourage successful practice. Yoga props and clothes are readily available on the Internet or in stores that sell sports equipment. We will explain some of what is available.

Keep in mind that many of the aids are extras. You don't have to purchase a lot of things in order to practice yoga, but some people will find that yoga equipment enhances their safety, increases their motivation, improves their practice, or adds to their overall enjoyment of yoga. Others may prefer the pure tradition with minimum additions. Let your own experience be your guide.

Yoga Props

Iyengar, true to his spirit of innovation, introduced a number of aids to enhance yoga learning and practice, and then manufacturers designed various products based on these original concepts. The main ones are mats, cushions, straps, blocks, and balls.

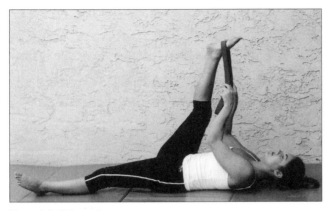

Figure 6-1: Using a strap

Yoga is performed on the floor. Traditionally, teachers recommend that you do the balancing, sitting, and lying down postures on a thin mat. Everyone should have a yoga mat for home practice. Today, safe, supportive yoga mats are being produced that also give you an optimal amount of softness. Mats also offer insulation from cold floors. Blankets and towels can also make sufficient mats; however, they tend to move and slip and bunch in a way that manufactured yoga mats do not.

Yoga mats are slightly sticky, providing a safe, nonslip surface for doing poses. Typically these mats are one-eighth of an inch thick and measure two feet wide by approximately six feet long. Another kind of mat rolls up like a sleeping bag and slides into a case, which then ties for easy carrying. These tend to be a little thicker, up to two inches, and are used for meditation or as a sleeping mat for retreats.

Cushions are useful for sitting poses and for easing into a more challenging position. You can use any thin pillow that is supportive without being too soft. Small cushions can be purchased from meditation supply stores.

Straps can be helpful when you are getting started, to begin the stretching process (Figure 6-1). For example, some beginners have difficulty bending forward in the seated forward stretch. A strap around the feet can help gently tug you forward with control, without going too far, too fast. More advanced students use straps to intensify their stretches and to move more deeply into postures.

Straps are generally six feet long, although they also come in eight- and nine-foot lengths. The width is from one inch, for narrow straps, to two inches. They are usually

Pillows, mats, straps, blocks, and balls are some of the typical yoga aids. Most schools will use mats, and many others will allow pillows. Straps, blocks, and balls are less common, but some people will find them to be invaluable tools to ease into stretching and strength building.

made with cotton and have a buckle to secure them, but release easily.

Blocks are lightweight but stable pieces of foam or wood, usually measuring about four inches thick by six inches wide and nine inches long. They are used to give support for many types of postures. You can sit on the block in seated positions, stand on it when practicing hamstring stretches, or use it to support your hands on the floor. Foam blocks are available with various levels of firmness, distinguished by color. Some have squared-off edges, and others have beveled edges. Wood blocks are usually birch, hollowed out to make them lightweight.

Yoga exercise balls are designed to help strengthen the lower back, abdomen, chest, and arms. They increase flexibility, tone, and range of motion. Balance and coordination are also improved. You can sit on the yoga ball, lie over it, or rest your feet on it when lying prone. Larger exercise balls are available for taller people, and smaller ones for shorter people.

Yoga Apparel

Most yoga teachers recommend that you set aside certain clothing for your yoga sessions. In this way, when you put on your yoga clothes, you will tend to feel like doing yoga. You can wear whatever is comfortable for a yoga session, but certain types of clothing work best. Clothes should allow ease of movement but should not get in your way when you bend or twist. For these reasons, nonbinding tops with loose-fitting pants are most popular. Clothes that restrict movement, such as blue jeans, should not be worn for yoga. Feet are usually bare to allow you to grip the floor well.

> The most important consideration in yoga apparel is ease of movement and comfort in wear. Yoga fashion can be fun to follow, so long as style doesn't get in the way of your practice.

Typically, women wear a tank top or T-shirt. Often the top has a built-in bra to give good support. Drawstring shorts, Capri leggings, tights, or pants that are nonbinding are commonly worn. Men usually wear either fitted shorts similar to bicycle shorts or drawstring pants and T-shirts or tank tops. You should wear natural fabrics, when possible, in keeping with yoga's preference for the unprocessed and organic. Materials such as natural cotton gauze let your skin breathe as you become warm from the workout.

Keep in mind that these clothing ideas are meant to be guidelines only. Wear clothing that is comfortable for you and makes you feel good about yourself.

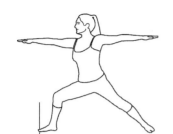

The mind must be directed toward itself.
—*Swami Nikhilananda*

YOGA CAN BE POSITIVE and health promoting. But, as with any physical activity, you must take certain precautions in order to be successful. Keep in mind some simple safety guidelines, and you will be able to enjoy the practice of yoga just as so many others have for many centuries.

Check with a Physician

Before you commence a new exercise program, check with your doctor or health-care professional. This is especially important if you have any chronic physical conditions such as high blood pressure, back or neck problems, arthritis, or heart disease. Depending on your doctor's recommendations, you may need to modify or eliminate some of the exercises in this book. Respect your body's needs. Cautions and limitations are given throughout the text, but there is no substitute for professional guidance. Use good sense in your individual situation.

After you have consulted your physician, use your own body reactions for additional feedback. If you pay attention to your sensations and interpret them correctly, your body will give you indications of what you can and cannot do. There is no benefit to be gained by pushing yourself too hard. Yoga works gradually. Be patient. Even the stiffest joints will become looser after regular, gentle practice.

Clear an Area

Once you have decided to try yoga at home, you will need to create a suitable space for doing it safely. Find a place where you can put your mat down. Clear away any furniture or objects around that area to create an open space at least five feet by eight feet. You need to be able to move freely without anything getting in your way.

> Creating a safe, comfortable area for your yoga practice will help to make your experience rewarding and safe. Most homes, even small apartments, can accommodate yoga practice with a few small modifications.

A carpeted or wooden floor surface are both fine to use. If you choose a wooden floor, place a yoga mat down to pad the surface. Place cushions in front of any furniture that is nearby to protect you in case you lose your balance during some postures. Make certain that all cables and extension cords are completely cleared away.

Yoga and Drugs

The practice of yoga involves being natural, which means avoiding anything artificial unless it is necessary for your health and well-being. Yogis believe that people can enhance their energy through healthy habits.

Yoga should not be performed after drinking coffee or taking stimulants. Also, do not perform yoga after drinking alcohol or taking other kinds of mood-altering substances.

Check with your doctor if you are taking medication to ensure that it is compatible with yoga practice. For example, there are medications that affect your balance, impair your concentration, or have other effects that are incompatible with yoga practice.

Keep Practice Slow

Yoga asanas are performed slowly and smoothly for the greatest benefits, so don't rush through your workout. Even the weight-loss exercises that are performed continuously at a slightly quicker pace should be done smoothly. In fact, doing the movements too quickly will diminish their benefit. The powerful effect that yoga can have comes from a slow and steady pace. The more advanced yogis move slowly and hold positions longer: This is a sign of skill in yoga. Even though the movements are slow, they can be demanding. The effects are subtle, but definite. If you are doing the weight-reduction routine in chapter 17, or if you join a power yoga class, you may move more quickly, but never sacrifice correct form. Moving too quickly may result in incorrect form, leading to possible injury. Sensing each movement helps you to move safely.

Be especially careful as you go into a pose and come out of it. Sometimes students think that the transitions are not really part of the asana, so they stop paying attention. Focused concentration during these moments of shifting position will help to keep your practice safe and productive.

Don't Ignore Your Limitations

Keep your personal limitations in mind. For example, during pregnancy, routines should be modified. Elderly people must also modify their routine to work with their bodies. Yoga offers advantages to athletes who may want to use yoga to enhance their skills. But even athletes should be careful when performing unfamiliar movements. Overweight and unfit individuals should carefully ease into the positions. Be gentle with yourself and you will make progress. Books geared to specific needs are available. Research your needs to devise the best routine to achieve the results you are looking for.

Don't Push Too Hard

When performing any of the yoga positions, go only as far as you can without pain. If you feel any pain, pull back to where you are comfortable. Your own sensations of pain are a signal to you that you may be risking injury, so don't force yourself into positions that hurt.

Some yoga routines can be vigorous, so it is important to pace yourself. If you notice your pulse rate increasing, stop and rest. Pay attention to how your body is being affected. With care, you will progress.

Safety during Pregnancy

You can practice yoga during pregnancy by modifying the routines. It is unwise to do a strenuous routine. Instead, substitute more meditation and breathing. Listen to your body, and feel what is comfortable and what is not. Always stop doing any asana that causes discomfort.

It's never too late to start a yoga program. Many of the great yoga gurus are in their eighties and older. The gentle movements, careful breathing exercises, and calming meditations will benefit people of all ages.

One important rule for pregnant women is to delete any asanas that are performed lying on your stomach, such as the locust, cobra, or bow. Yoga includes so many different kinds of asanas that you will find plenty of positions that do not put any stress on the abdominal region.

Modify some of the other poses to make them more comfortable for you and your baby. For example, when leaning back in the sun salutation, place your hands behind your back at your waist, to brace yourself. When you go down to the floor, keep your abdomen raised off the ground, letting your arms and legs support you. When lying on your back for leg raises, lift one leg at a time. Don't do the double leg raise.

Several seated positions can be modified for pregnancy. For seated forward stretches, straddle your legs apart so that you make space for your stomach when you bend forward. Seated twists can also be adapted. Sit in an easy pose and place your left hand on the outside of your right knee, and your right hand on the floor behind you. Look to the right. You will notice that this twist gives you a good stretch without interfering with the baby.

Use common sense and don't press, push, or overly stretch your abdominal area. Then you will enjoy the benefits of calmness, flexibility, strength, and fitness that yoga can bring you. Your baby responds to your feelings and moods. When you are calm and tranquil, so is your baby! The safety and well-being of your little one can be enhanced by finding your own calm center. So practice meditation and pranayama regularly.

Yoga Later in Life

Yoga can be started later in life or continued on into old age if you take certain precautions. Careful yoga practice may help you sleep better. You may find that you have more energy and feel stronger and more flexible.

One of the most important guidelines is: Don't push too hard or too fast. If you feel yourself getting out of breath, lie down in savasana pose until you feel relaxed. Stretch only as far as you can go comfortably. You will find that by slow, steady effort you will begin to loosen up.

Find the best time of day to practice. Some people are looser and more energetic in the morning but get stiff and tired later. Others feel most alert and comfortable later in the day. You probably know your own patterns. Use them to your advantage and start doing yoga during your peak times. Eventually you will be able to do it at varied times if you want.

Use a chair if you can't sit comfortably on the floor. Many of the poses can be done from a chair, such as forward bends, twists, and leg raises. People who want to sit on the floor should sit on a pillow to take the strain off the legs.

Warm up carefully when you begin, and also be sure to stretch out briefly when you finish. As people get older, warming up and warming down become even more important, although people of all ages will benefit from warming up and down. Try to warm up every part of your body. This includes wrists, ankles, and neck.

Modify asanas to fit your capabilities. For example, with leg raises, just raise one leg at a time. Use aids such as blocks, pillows, or chairs to help modify your position. For example, when doing a forward bend, bend only partway and grip a sturdy chair back. Even a small movement can be a beginning on a path to more vigorous and comfortable living.

Practice pranayama and meditation regularly. The awareness that you gain can be helpful throughout your day.

Recovering from Illness

If you are convalescing from an illness or recovering from an injury, you can also do a little bit of yoga to help you recover more quickly. Many of the yoga asanas can be done in bed, along with breathing and meditation. Modify the lying-down positions to fit your abilities. Don't push yourself too hard. If you feel dizzy, stop and meditate. Your endurance may be lower than normal, so your exercise routine may need to be shortened considerably. Even a few minutes a day may help to stimulate your immune system to heal you more quickly. Be sure to do some pranayama and meditation, as these tools can be very helpful.

Yoga can be practiced by all kinds of people during all phases of life, as long as certain safety precautions are taken and careful modifications are made. Then anyone can enjoy the benefits of yoga without harm.

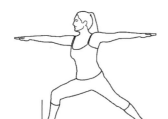

chapter 8

preparing for your first session

*Through becoming conscious we have been driven out of paradise,
through consciousness we can come back to paradise.*
—Heinrich Jacoby

THE PRACTICE OF YOGA teaches you how to listen, feel, and sense. It gently and gradually points you back to the fundamentals of breathing, sitting, standing, and moving. From this firm foundation, everything in life becomes easier and more natural. Attending to the inside can make a difference on the outside. Self-awareness grounds you in your life and your world, so that you can intuitively know what to do and have the self-discipline to do it. So if you approach your yoga practice with a receptive, open awareness, you enrich the quality of everyday living.

First Glimpse

Try this exercise to help you orient your mind to yoga. Your mental attitude is very important.

Pick a time when you are not busy and do not have any immediate demands on your time. Sit down in a quiet place. Stay quiet for a moment, without thinking about what you should be doing next. Just stay with right now, in this moment.

Try turning your attention to your sensations. What do you feel from the chair or bench, as you sit? Is the surface soft or hard? Do you sink into a pillow, or does the chair press against your back and seat? Can you allow yourself to sit in the chair, rather than on it? What does the temperature of the air feel like? Is it warm or cool?

Pay attention to what you sense from your body. For example, notice your breathing. Can you be aware of the air coming in and going out? Notice your muscles. Do you feel tension in any particular muscle area?

Now stand up slowly. Notice the movement as you do so. Which muscles are involved, and how do you balance? Can you move smoothly without hurrying?

The time and place for yoga are when and where you make them. Make yoga compatible with your lifestyle and you will find yourself doing yoga naturally and regularly.

These are some of the sensory details, the qualities, that you will pay attention to as you perform yoga postures. The focused intensity of attention that you bring to yoga is a major part of successful practice. If you can learn to apply this kind of attention to yourself when you perform yoga, your practice will be immensely enriched. The chapters that follow will guide you in specific ways to focus on your experience as you learn the yoga basics: breathing, postures, and meditation.

Where and When to Practice at Home

If you do yoga at home, you will need a particular place. Find an area of the house for doing yoga that has enough space for you to be able to move around without bumping into furniture or walls. Bring a mat and spread it on the floor to give you a little bit of cushioning.

Pick a time when you will be undisturbed for at least thirty minutes. When you are first beginning, half an hour is long enough. You probably will gradually increase the amount of time you devote to practice. Most regular yoga classes are at least an hour or an hour and a half long; but allow your own body to guide you. No matter what length of time you choose to devote to yoga, make sure that your routine always includes warmups, a series of postures (asanas), breathing (pranayama), and meditation. So if you decide to shorten your workout, don't delete any category, just do less of each one.

Yoga should be performed on an empty stomach. The usual rule is to schedule your practice for three or four hours after eating. If necessary, eat a light snack an hour or so before.

Keep the safety guidelines in mind, as described in chapter 7: Don't do anything that doesn't feel good. Don't move too quickly, and above all, never push yourself too far. Ahimsa also applies to you, not just to others—don't harm yourself.

Warmup Exercises

Before you engage in the postures themselves, it is important to warm up your body. You will derive the most benefit from warmups by paying close attention to the movements as you perform them. Whenever you do warmups, be sure to bring your attention to them as well.

Perform these simple warmup exercises before you begin any of the yoga routines in this book. Also do them before trying the individual asanas in Part III.

When you begin to stretch, start from wherever you are. Don't try to push beyond what is comfortable. Do the exercises slowly, without straining. You will make progress if you practice carefully and gradually. You will enjoy the benefits that you can achieve from gentle, sensitive stretching.

Upward Stretch

Begin by standing upright, feet together. Raise your open hands overhead, extending your fingers, and stretch your arms gently upward as you inhale. Let your ribcage lift as your whole body extends up a bit, and then exhale while you let your arms bend at the elbows and slowly sink back to your sides. Repeat several times.

Self-awareness is the gateway to wisdom. We all have the capacity to be enlightened. Begin with an inward glance, and a world of possibilities opens up to you.

Head Roll

Keep your arms resting down at your sides. Limber your neck muscles and upper spine by tilting your head sideways, so that your right ear moves closer to your right shoulder. Then gently roll your head forward, bringing your chin toward your chest. Continue by moving your head around to the left, so that your left ear moves toward your left shoulder, then let your head tilt back slightly. Continue to roll your head around in a circle in this way, three times and then repeat in reverse.

Shoulder Roll

Keep your arms down at your sides. Lift your shoulders slightly and gently roll them forward, up, back, and down. Continue to roll your shoulders around, three times in one direction and then three times in the reverse direction. This exercise helps to relieve tension from sitting long hours at a desk.

Though they are sometimes ignored, careful warmups of the neck and shoulders will not only help them to become stronger and more flexible, but will also make them feel more comfortable throughout your day.

Forward Bend

Inhale as you raise your arms up over your head again, and then slowly lower your body forward. Let your arms hang down toward the floor, and let your head relax. Do not strain beyond a comfortable forward bend. Raise and lower three times.

Bent Elbow Twist

Move your legs about a foot apart and bend your arms, raising them to shoulder height. Place one hand on top of the other and inhale, as you stand comfortably upright. Then gently pivot your arms around to the right, allowing your body to stretch around too, as you exhale. Come back to center and inhale, and then pivot to the left for a stretch on the other side as you exhale again. Repeat three times on each side.

Just as an automobile needs to be warmed up before it runs optimally, you should always give yourself a few minutes of preliminary stretches to warm up your body before you begin your yoga routine.

Side Stretch

Now place your legs about two shoulder widths apart, with your feet facing straight ahead. Inhale as you extend your arms out sideways from your shoulders, holding them parallel to the floor. Then extend your right hand overhead while exhaling, and lean over sideways to the left, to give you a gentle side stretch. Keep your legs straight. Lower your arm back to extend outwards as you return to an upright position, facing front, and inhale. Then exhale as you raise your left arm overhead and then stretch to the other side. Don't push too hard or stretch too deeply on either side. Keep in mind that you are just trying to limber up and warm up your muscles.

Chest Stretch

Return to standing upright with legs together and clasp your hands behind your back, with arms extending downward. Press your shoulder blades toward each other as you press your hands together and inhale. Then relax your shoulders and arms as you exhale. Repeat three times.

People with any knee problems can modify the lower back stretch to protect the knees. To do this, hold your legs behind the knees as you pull gently. Bend the kneed a little if necessary.

Lower Back Stretch

Lie on the floor on your back and inhale. Then bring your knees up toward your chest as you exhale. Hold your legs below the knees and pull gently, allowing a light stretch of your lower back. Release your legs and inhale again. Then repeat two more times.

Leg Swing

Limber up your legs by gently swinging your left leg forward and then back, slowly and carefully. Repeat with the right leg. You can keep your hands on your hips or hold on to a stable chair back, counter, or wall, if you feel unsteady. Keep the swings controlled, relaxed, and easy. Repeat three or four times on each side as you breathe normally.

Now you are ready to begin. Familiarize yourself with the elements of yoga in part 3: postures, breathing, and meditation. Then begin with the first routine in part 4, the sun salutation, in chapter 14. You can also start with the relaxing routine in chapter 15. As you become more familiar with the postures, try one of the other routines, especially if it seems appropriate for a specific goal you have in mind. But keep an open mind! Although you may wish to accomplish concrete goals, you will also enjoy some of the more intangible mental and spiritual rewards of yoga practice.

part 3
elements

THE FUNDAMENTAL ELEMENTS of a yoga workout are postures (asanas), breathing (pranayama), and meditation. Breathing and concentration should always be part of each yoga posture. Concentrated attention helps you to move, breathe, and focus in the correct way. These practices are the elements of yoga.

The unity of yoga, achieved by linking body, mind, and spirit, is truly expressed in every posture you do, every breath you take, and every thought you have during practice. Yoga brings together all these elements, uniting mind and body consciously. This unified approach to practice can extend into your everyday life. Mind, body, and spirit can work together naturally, as you have trained them to do.

The next five chapters present the basic yoga elements. Familiarize yourself with the asana postures, pranayama breathing exercises, and meditations presented in part 3. These basic elements, along with additional variations, are in the routines given in part 4.

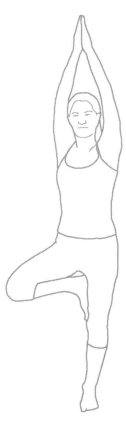

standing and balancing asanas

Asanas must have the dual qualities of alertness and relaxation. . . .
When these principles are correctly followed, asana practice will help
a person endure and even minimize the external influences on the
body such as age, climate, diet, and work.
—The Yoga Sutras of Patanjali

YOGA CAN BE DONE successfully at various levels. Yoga practice starts with what a person can do easily and comfortably, without strain. Don't worry if you can't do the postures perfectly, or if you have an injury that prevents certain movements. By working within or around limitations, you can still make progress. Yoga is a practice of intense personal focus—if you are practicing with your full intention, you are doing the best anyone can do. Even if barely in the asana, you are embarking on the yoga path.

Patanjali's *Yoga Sutras* describe two qualities that are important to develop when performing asanas: *sthira*, alertness, and *sukha*, relaxation. "These qualities can be achieved by recognizing and observing the reactions of the body and the breath to the various postures that comprise asana practice. Once known, these reactions can be controlled step-by-step." (Patanjali, in Desikachar 1995, p. 180) Learning to be both alert and relaxed while performing the asanas may have a positive effect that

Mind and body work together as you learn to combine the elements of yoga: breathing, asanas, and meditation. The unifying of movement, breath, and thought has a profound effect that makes yoga much more than a simple exercise regime.

carries over into everyday life. The movements are performed with awareness, and at the same time are performed without tension. Alertness and relaxation may not seem to go together, because being alert might seem to require a forced effort. But in yoga, the goal is to be able to approach each posture without forcing, with a naturally attuned awareness that is also calm. In this way, more can be accomplished. Over time, you will develop the ability to sustain both states of mind together, by combining all the elements of yoga: breathing, meditation, and asanas.

Yoga practice moves your body in every direction and from different starting points, giving you a balanced workout. As such, asanas can be divided into categories: standing, lying prone, inverted, and sitting. This way of thinking about poses is useful in helping you to insure that your routine includes each type of movement for an all-body effect.

Asanas involve more than simply moving the body into a posture and holding it there. Each asana has three aspects: moving into the pose, holding the pose, and then coming out of it again. The movement into the pose, the holding, and then the movement out of the pose should be performed smoothly, calmly, without rushing, and with balance and poise. Even when performing postures quickly for a more vigorous workout, maintain smoothness and control without straining.

Asanas can be divided into several basic categories: standing, lying prone, inverted, sitting. These categories include forward bends, backward bends, twists, and balancing. More advanced postures often combine two or more of these basic movements into position and out of position. The gentle, gradual practice of these traditional asanas, combined with breathing exercises and meditation, confers benefits on many levels. Greater flexibility, strength, and endurance are some of the physical returns from regular practice.

Standing Asanas

Routines usually begin with standing asanas. Much of our life is spent standing on our two feet. We balance upright and walk from the standing position. Our spine keeps us upright, giving us support. We gauge where we are and orient ourselves perceptually from our height. And so it is logical that standing asanas are an important part of yoga.

Yoga exercises done standing up will help you in many ways. The standing postures build strength, coordination, and flexibility. Improved body alignment and poise develop a feeling of well-being and comfort. Daily activities become easier and more energetic.

The standing asana elements consist of bending forward, bending backward, and twisting, to help you become more flexible. You will also gain strength from these positions. The muscles on both sides of the spine are exercised by these forward, backward, and twisting positions.

Another primary benefit of asanas in general is balance and centering. The standing asanas—particularly positions balanced on one leg—work on these skills directly. You learn how to find your center and keep it. As you perform these postures, first on one side and then on the other, you may notice that the two sides of your body are different. Most people find that positions are easier on one side than on the other. In fact, people often favor one side more than the other. Yoga works both sides equally, which helps develop the weaker side. By using both sides of the body, you also stimulate the two hemispheres of the brain. Eventually, mind and body become balanced and integrated, working together for optimal functioning.

Yoga helps us to develop a strong and balanced stance. From this firm base, all of life's movements become easier and more comfortable.

Standing postures can be physically demanding, so it is important to ease into them carefully. As you go into a standing posture—or any yoga posture for that matter—you can always make little adjustments, to improve the correctness of your position, to relax more, to breathe more fully, or to discover more comfort. Here is where feedback from a teacher or experienced practitioner may help. Working out with a friend or partner may also be useful. Sometimes a mirror may help provide feedback. If you are doing yoga alone at home, be aware of your body and work sensitively with it.

Use special care with certain areas. The neck, lower back, and knees are three sensitive areas of the body that should be carefully protected when doing standing postures. Try to keep your neck as relaxed as possible, lengthening it without straining. Do the same with the lower back region: try to lengthen it without overstretching. The knee joints are easily injured, but with correct positioning, the muscles and ligaments surrounding the knees can help to protect them. Bend your knees carefully, and try to keep the forward one over the center of your foot. Let your knee bend like a hinge, and do not twist it for added rotation. When standing, if you do rotate your knee, let the movement originate from the hip joint, not the foot.

Keep your breathing coordinated with your movements. Breathing is one of the keys to successful practice. It helps you to keep your motions fluid and circular rather than stiff or abrupt. Keep relaxing as you go, and in time your body will respond.

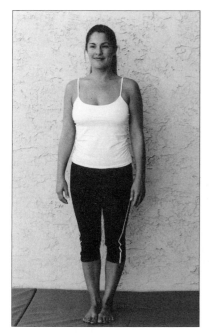

Figure 9-1: Mountain pose

Mountain Pose, Tadasana

A fundamental position for standing asanas is standing aligned, and with awareness. You will begin and end many series with the mountain pose. People often neglect their posture, and then find themselves with habits that can cause aches, pains, and fatigue. Poor posture often forces you to fight against gravity, thereby wasting your energy. When you can stand straight with your feet firmly on the ground, legs under you, spine straight, and head centered, gravity becomes your ally. Alignment is natural, and standing becomes effortless.

Stand with feet together, ankles touching, and arms at your sides. Stand up straight, yet be relaxed. Keep your shoulders from slumping, and don't let your back hunch (Figure 9-1).

Let your weight be evenly balanced between your two feet, and balanced front to back. If the balance point is not readily apparent, close your eyes. Rock very gently from side to side, and feel the balance point shifting from one leg to the other. You will notice a position in which balance is effortless,

Mountains are symbolic of formidable power and mystical wisdom. When you can develop a well-balanced mountain pose, you draw strength from the ground and reach toward the heavens.

and weight is shared exactly by both legs. Stand for a moment or two as you sense this point. Next, try rocking very slightly forward and back. You will feel your muscles tighten up as you shift forward and backward. Notice the point in the middle where your muscles relax. Find the place between side to side and forward and back where you are most relaxed and balanced, aligned with gravity. Now with your body standing comfortably straight, you are firm, like a mountain.

Chest Expansion Pose

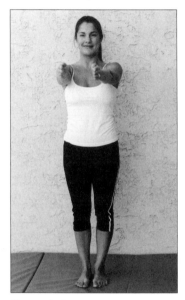
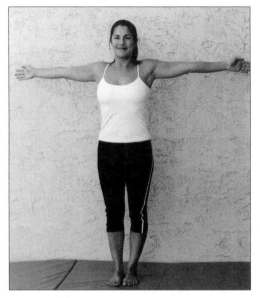

Figure 9-2: Chest expansion, first part   Figure 9-3: Chest expansion, second part

Learning to open up your chest and allow the air to flow freely through your lungs is fundamental. As breathing capacity expands, your energy level will rise and you will become healthier. You can begin this ongoing process by expanding your chest.

Stand in the mountain pose and extend your arms out directly in front of you as you exhale (Figure 9-2). Maintain your balance and let your arms swing around behind you, parallel to the floor, while you inhale. Let the air fill your lungs fully as you allow your chest to expand (Figure 9-3). Exhale as you circle your hands back around to the front. Repeat this pattern several times, coordinating your breathing with the movement.

Bending Asanas

The health and flexibility of the back are important. Many yoga asanas include different types of bends with specific instructions. Correct bending can strengthen and loosen the spine, which has a positive effect on the back.

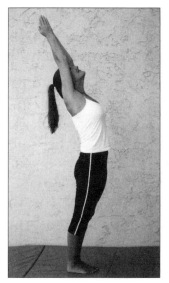

Figure 9-4: Sun pose, first part

Standing Sun Pose

One of the fundamental yoga asanas for bending is the sun pose. It is usually done standing, but can be modified for sitting on the floor, or even in a chair. This posture is part of a larger sun salutation routine in part 4.

The sun pose incorporates the body's natural forward and backward bending abilities to help improve digestion and circulation. It exercises the heart and lungs, and the backs of the legs. The muscles around the spine are also strengthened and limbered.

Begin standing with your feet together and arms down at your sides, in the mountain pose. Exhale

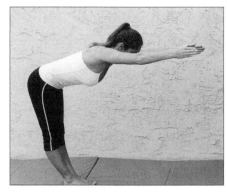

Figure 9-5: Sun pose, second part

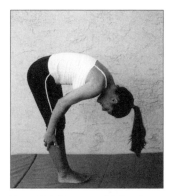

Figure 9-6: Sun pose, third part

completely. Then, begin inhaling as you circle your arms out and up above your head until your palms touch each other. Arch slightly backward as you look up and finish inhaling (Figure 9-4). Hold for a moment, and then breathe out and bend forward from the waist. Try to keep your back relatively straight for as long as possible as you bend all the way down (Figure 9-5). Keep your head tucked between your arms while exhaling. Let your hands hang down toward the floor. Grasp the back of your legs as far down as comfortable, while keeping your legs relatively straight, and gently pull yourself down (Figure 9-6). Back off from where it begins to hurt. Be careful not to pull your muscles. Beginners may bend their knees a little at first, eventually keeping them straight. It may take repeated tries, depending on your flexibility. Let your arms bend at the elbows as you hold; this will help to ensure that you are using your arms to pull you down, not your back.

As people grow older they may not bend their bodies very often. Yoga encourages careful bending to help keep the body fit and elastic.

Hold for a few seconds at the bottom of your exhale, and then let go of your legs and slowly return to the standing position. This exercise may be repeated several times in a row.

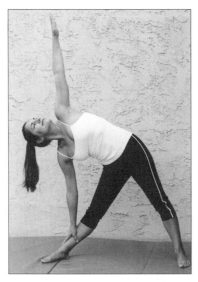

Figure 9-7: Triangle pose

Triangle, Trikonasana

The triangle pose is a sideways bend. This posture is very helpful for trimming the waistline and adding more strength and flexibility to the midsection, while toning the muscles around the spine. It also increases circulation to the arms.

Begin with your legs several feet apart and your feet facing forward. Raise your arms out sideways to shoulder height with hands open, palms facing downward, as you inhale. Slowly bend to the left, keeping your arms stretched out, and begin exhaling. Let your left arm and shoulder rotate down so your left hand can slide down along the side of the left knee, or as low as you can comfortably go, while keeping the right arm extended overhead. The open right hand points straight up overhead. Keep your legs relatively straight. Look up toward your raised hand and feel the stretch in your right side (Figure 9-7). Slowly straighten up, while inhaling again, and return to the starting position. Repeat the same motions on the other side.

Twisting Asanas

A healthy back can move in many directions. Twisting motions add flexibility to the lower back and waist. Several asanas help to develop mobility of the lower back through carefully controlled twisting motions.

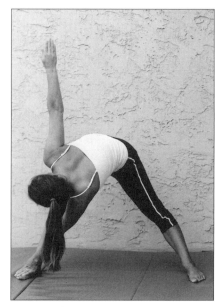

Figure 9-8: Twisting triangle

Twisting Triangle, Trikonasana Parivritta

The triangle posture can be varied to add a twisting stretch. This position will stretch your spine, while also helping to tone your waist.

To perform the twisting triangle, place yourself in the opening position of the triangle posture, with feet wide apart. Inhale as you raise and extend your arms straight out from your sides so that they are parallel to the floor, palms facing down. Exhale as you bend forward toward your right leg, grasping the outside of your right ankle with your left hand. You may need to take hold higher up on your leg, if you can't reach your ankle. As you take hold of your leg, let your open right hand point straight up, with fingers loosely extended. Look up at your raised hand to increase the stretch, keeping your knees straight (Figure 9-8). Hold for a few seconds, and then return to the standing position as you slowly inhale. Repeat on the left side, exhaling slowly as you go down, and inhaling as you stand up.

Archer Pose

The archer pose simulates holding and pulling a large bow, as in archery. It teaches you to focus your attention on your posture and balance, while gently twisting your upper body. It offers a good upper-body stretch while helping improve concentration.

Begin with your right foot directly

Yoga draws on the stability of the triangle, a three-sided geometric figure. By moving your body into this asana, you can incorporate the triangle's stability to help you enhance flexibility and strength.

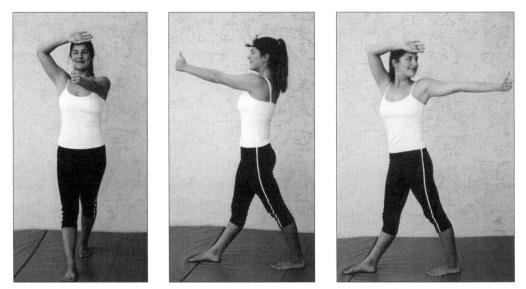

Figure 9-9: Archer pose, front view   Figure 9-10: Archer pose, first part   Figure 9-11: Archer pose, second part

in front of your left, toes pointing straight ahead, as though standing on a narrow balance beam. If you are a beginner, you may want to allow your stance to be a bit wider, with feet farther apart, until you get accustomed to the posture. Pretend that you are holding a large bow. Extend your left arm out straight ahead with the fist closed, as if holding the bow. Place the back of your right hand on your forehead in a loose fist, as if holding the string. Look straight ahead at your extended left hand, and inhale (Figures 9-9 and 9-10). Then slowly begin exhaling while turning toward the right, keeping your arms positioned, and gazing at your extended thumb (Figure 9-11). Twist your upper body back as far as you comfortably can, and hold for a few seconds. Inhale as you gently untwist to face front again. Switch position by placing the left foot forward, with the right arm holding the imaginary bow extended in front and the right arm bent. Now repeat the movements, twisting to the other side.

Yoga uses many metaphors for the asanas. Archery was a commonly practiced sport and art of ancient times. The movements of drawing a bow can become a resource for you today as it did for so many people through the ages.

Balancing Asanas

Balancing is an important component of yoga asanas. When you are trying to balance, your attention is automatically drawn to the task. Almost effortlessly, your mind is concentrated where it needs to be. So these exercises not only train your body to balance, but also indirectly train you to focus, an important lesson in yoga. When your mind and body work together as one, you will be surprised at how much more effective you will be in whatever you do.

> **B**alance can be symbolic of many things. For example, we think of balancing our lives between work and play, between inner and outer, between individual needs and the needs of the world. Finding balance is intuitive and can be developed as you turn your attention to it.

Warrior Pose, Virabhadrasana

The warrior pose has similarities to a martial arts front stance, with some variation. Like a martial arts stance, the warrior pose is a powerful, stable position. It requires careful balance, as it also develops strength. The warrior pose will develop the muscles in your feet and arches, your legs, abdomen, and shoulders. It offers a good stretch for the chest and enhances circulation throughout the body. It is considered one of the best exercises for firming the calf, thigh, and trunk muscles.

Step out to leave a fairly wide distance between your feet, approximately three feet apart, depending upon how long your legs are. You can place the outer edge of your back foot against a wall to keep you more stable. Bend your front knee, keeping the lower leg perpendicular to the floor, and the thigh parallel to the floor, so that the bent leg forms as close to a 90-degree angle as possible. Beginners should ease into this with less of a bend. Keep your hips on a level plane. Spread your two arms out from your sides, parallel to the floor, with fingers held together and pointing straight out. Turn your head to face the bent forward leg, while keeping your neck and back straight. Lift your chest, stretching out through your hands and fingers. Hold the position while continuing to breathe in and out for a few seconds (Figure 9-12). Then repeat on the other side.

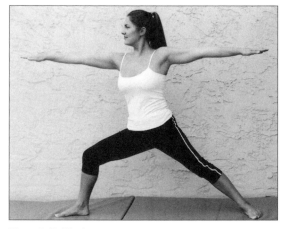

Figure 9-12: Warrior pose

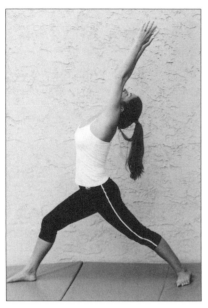

Figure 9-13: Warrior pose II

Warrior Pose II

This pose is a lunging position. It loosens and strengthens the shoulders and chest, while also strengthening the trunk and legs. The ribcage is raised, allowing more air to flow and energy to rise.

Step out as in the first warrior pose, with your feet approximately three to four feet apart, keeping your right leg straight as you exhale. This time, however, turn your chest and torso to the right so that your whole body faces squarely right—a position very similar to the martial arts front stance. You may let the back foot pivot diagonally to take strain off your knees. Then begin to inhale as you bend your front knee. As your knee bends, raise your arms straight over your head with palms facing forward, and arch back gently with the inhale. Pause when your lower leg is close to perpendicular to the ground directly over the foot and your upper leg is nearly parallel to the ground. Hold the position for several breaths (Figure 9-13). Inhale while straightening your leading leg, and then, while exhaling, lower your arms and bring your front foot back to meet the back one. Yoga includes many different types of lunges with different hand positions and varying angles of the upper body. For example, a variation of this lunging motion is incorporated into the sun salutation routine included in part 4.

According to martial arts legends, warriors were honorable people who fought for justice. They trained to endure harsh conditions and learned to perform amazing feats of strength and agility. Yoga draws upon the best qualities of the warrior through the warrior positions.

Tree Pose, Vrikshasana

The tree pose is a classic yoga exercise that requires you to balance on one foot. With practice you will learn to feel centered and at ease on one leg. Yogis believe that balancing enhances body awareness, since successful balance requires your mind to be focused on your action.

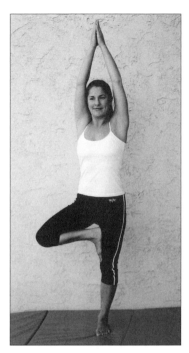

Figure 9-14: Tree pose

To perform this asana, pick a spot at eye level directly in front of you, to gaze at. This will make it easier to keep your head upright and straight. Raise your right leg and place your right foot, toes pointing down, as high on the inside of your left leg as you can, while remaining in balance. Press the foot inwards against the left thigh. Open the hip of the bent knee, but don't let your other hip turn in. You can prevent any twisting by tightening the buttocks muscles. When you feel stable, exhale completely. Then raise your arms straight overhead and bring your palms together. Extend your body upwards as you balance on one leg. Breathe normally and comfortably, in and out, for ten to thirty seconds. Keep looking at the spot you chose to gaze at, maintaining relaxed breathing (Figure 9-14). Repeat the exercise with the other leg raised.

Beginners might find that at first they cannot balance. You can ease into this exercise by standing next to a sturdy chair or a wall and supporting yourself with one hand. Raise your leg into position as instructed, letting the free hand rise overhead. Keep your breathing relaxed while performing the posture. Repeat on the other side.

Study a tree in your environment. Notice how the trunk is rooted in the ground and the branches reach outward to the sky. Sense how the tree is in balance with gravity. When you perform the tree posture, draw on your image of the tree to root your leg and allow your arms to reach for the sky in balance with gravity.

Dancer Pose

The dancer pose is another fundamental balancing pose that strengthens while enhancing flexibility and concentration. It builds the lower back and loosens the upper back. It also limbers up the legs, hips, and thighs. Ankles and feet are strengthened. The chest muscles are opened up, allowing for deeper breathing.

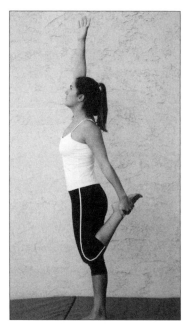

Figure 9-15: Dancer pose

To perform the dancer pose, stand straight with your feet together, looking straight ahead. Bend your left leg at the knee so that your left foot is directly behind you, and grasp your left foot or ankle with your left hand. Gently pull up and back, without straining, as you inhale. Stretch upwards with your right hand, keeping your back straight and aligned (Figure 9-15). Lean forward slightly, and you will feel a little more of a stretch in your thigh. Keep your stomach muscles relaxed and breathe comfortably in and out for ten to twenty seconds. Release, and perform the position on the other side.

Beginners can use a support to gradually transition into this posture. Stand behind a stable chair or near a wall and hold on as you raise and then grasp your rear leg. If you can balance well, try it without the support, and raise your arm overhead.

Keep working on doing these postures until you are familiar with what they are and how, generally, to perform them. You will perfect each posture over time, when you do them as part of your regular routine.

Dancers are graceful and fluid in their movements. The dancer pose can enhance your grace and poise. Move slowly and enjoy the stretch.

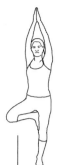

chapter 10

lying prone and
inverted asanas

To know ourselves means to know our relationship
with the world—not only with the world of ideas and people,
but also with nature, with the things we possess.
That is our life—life being relationship to the whole.
—J. Krishnamurti

L IFE IS ALWAYS in relationship to the whole. As we saw in the last chapter, when you are standing, there is a relationship to gravity, to the ground you stand on, and to your balance. You can explore another dimension of these relationships through the practice of lying prone and inverted asanas. People can learn about themselves through their relationships with the world around them.

Yoga uses all the basic positions for postures: standing, sitting, and lying prone. The exercises for lying down are usually performed on a thin mat on the floor. Try to avoid an overly soft surface. Yoga mats are designed with the correct hardness.

When you are lying down, there is a relationship to the supporting surface. Many of the prone and inverted asanas can be performed more easily than the others, because of the support given by the floor. These postures include forward, backward, and twisting stretches, as do the standing and sitting postures. But because of the support from the floor, you will be able to work out different areas in new ways.

Yoga can teach you how to relax completely. When you are lying prone, you learn how to let go of all unnecessary tension and breathe comfortably. This ability to let go can help you to sleep more deeply at night and carry less tension in the day.

Rest Asanas

Several of the classic prone postures can be used to relax, for rest between asanas or for deep relaxation at times during the day. Savasana and crocodile poses can relax the body from head to foot.

Corpse Pose, Savasana

The savasana pose can help rejuvenate and revitalize you. Being very restful, the savasana pose can also bring about a feeling of well-being.

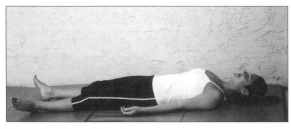

Figure 10-1: Corpse Pose, Savasana

Lie down on your back on the floor with legs extended and arms at your side, palms facing up. Let your feet move apart and rotate outwards slightly. Close your eyes. Breathe comfortably (Figure 10-1). Scan your body with your attention, and let go of any unnecessary tensions. People often hold extra tensions in the muscles of the face, stomach, neck, shoulders, and back, so let them go. Try to relax as deeply as you can. Rest in this position for a few minutes.

If you feel tightness in your lower back in this asana, you can modify the position by raising your knees while leaving your feet flat on the floor. You

---

Body awareness is one of the pathways to deeper relaxation. Turn your attention to your body as you lie in savasana. Let go of extra tension in your muscles and allow your breathing to be relaxed.

---

may want to put a pillow under your knees and let your legs extend comfortably. This tends to let the lower back flatten, allowing it to relax very deeply. As you feel the back muscles let go, you may be able to extend your legs flat into the corpse pose. If not, use the modified position to allow yourself to relax when needed.

Crocodile Pose, Makarasana

The crocodile pose is also a relaxation posture, performed lying on your stomach. According to Indian folklore, the crocodile is considered one of nature's

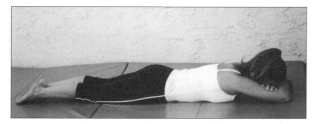

Figure 10-2: Crocodile pose, Makarasana

most extraordinary creatures because it can be comfortable on the earth as well as in the water. Thus this pose symbolizes the ability to be fully relaxed under any circumstance.

The crocodile pose can be helpful to the digestive system, massaging the abdomen slightly. Some people may find this pose more comfortable than savasana. If so, use this instead for deep relaxing.

Lie face down on the floor with your chin touching the ground and your hands at your sides. Let your legs stretch apart at a comfortable distance, wit' your heels facing in and toes pointing out. Bend one arm to make a res* place for your forehead, placing the hand on your opposite shoulder, fc

---

Use your awareness to help you relax in crocodile pose. Learning to relax fully in this pose may generalize to your sleeping position, giving you a more restful and rejuvenating night's sleep.

---

a triangle. Let the other hand come across your body at shoulder level and grasp the opposite side between the shoulder and the elbow. This position keeps your arms from moving as you totally relax. Once you are in position, let your body relax completely. Gently breathe in and out as you let go of any unnecessary tensions. Try to inhale and exhale for approximately the same length of time. Remain relaxed in this position for approximately one minute (Figure 10-2).

Knee Squeeze or Wind Relieving

This position rests the back as it gently lengthens the lower back muscles. It also relaxes the hips, improves circulation in the pelvic region, and helps digestion. The knee squeeze can be very relaxing after a yoga workout. You can extend this restful position into an exercise to tone the back and stomach.

Begin with the single knee squeeze to warm up. Rest on your back with arms extended overhead on the floor, and legs extended comfortably. Exhale.

PRATT & LAMBERT
Vert Serein
Serene Green
520©

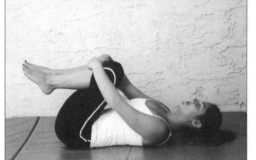

Figure 10-3: Knee squeezing, first part

Figure 10-4: Knee squeezing, second part

Then inhale when ready. As you begin to inhale, bend your left knee up and in toward your body, as you grasp the leg with your arms below the knee. You may prefer to grasp your leg behind the knee rather than over the knee. Lightly pull your knee in toward your chest as you exhale. Then hold for a few seconds as you breathe in and out, relaxing. Slowly release and extend your leg as you inhale. Then repeat with the other leg.

For the double knee squeeze, perform as before, only raise both knees together, then grasp both together, hold (Figure 10-3), and then release. Again, you may prefer to grasp behind your legs below the knees for less strain or a different stretching angle. Carefully coordinate the movements with your breathing, inhaling when your arms are extended overhead, exhaling as you bring your knees in and squeeze, and then inhaling again when you release and stretch out.

Yoga adds flexibility to your back. The knee squeeze positions are a gentle way to help the process of releasing tension in the back.

To perform this as an exercise that will gently massage your digestive system and work out your stomach muscles, begin by performing the single leg version. When your leg is raised and held, bring your head up off the ground, raising your chin toward your knee, exhale deeply as you squeeze, and then release. Repeat with each leg, and then perform with both legs up (Figure 10-4). You will feel a light contraction in your midsection. With both legs up you can also add a relaxing rocking motion to end the exercise. Rock gently, forward and backward and side to side, to lightly massage your back. Try to breathe comfortably as you rock, relaxing as deeply as possible.

Limbering and Strengthening Asanas

Many of the prone asanas will build strength and flexibility. The group that follows consists of classic postures used in most forms of yoga.

> **A** strong and flexible back is the foundation for a strong and flexible body. Yoga routines always include a number of asanas that build strength and enhance flexibility in the back and spine. The benefits are long lasting and generalize to the whole body.

Cobra Pose, Bhujangasana

The cobra pose is one of the core yoga asanas, incorporated into many routines, including the sun salutation (part 4). It is especially helpful for people who spend time sitting somewhat immobile at a desk or computer. The cobra pose helps to unlock the upper body, stretching and strengthening the spine, shoulders, and neck, as it sends blood circulating into these areas.

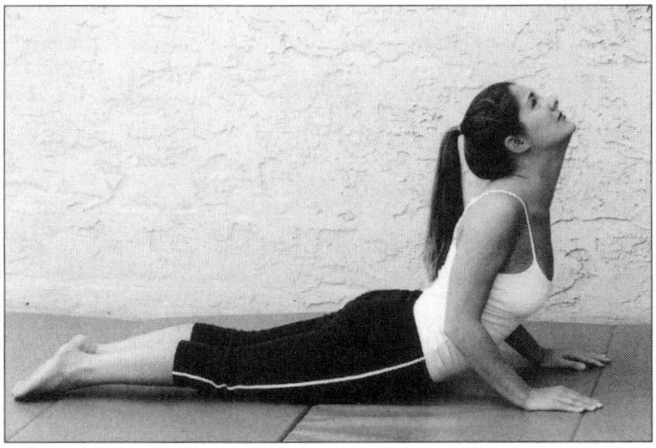

Figure 10-5: Cobra pose

The cobra pose draws upon the spirit of a cobra: With flexibility and strength, the cobra curls powerfully. Although the cobra pose may seem to resemble a push-up, the lower body and hips are pressed to the ground. Like a push-up, the cobra pose does strengthen the upper body somewhat, but unlike a push-up, this pose exercises and stretches the back through slow, sensitive movement. Never be sudden or forceful with this asana.

Lie down on your stomach with your legs together and your palms flat on the floor under your shoulders, your elbows held in close to your sides, and your forehead resting on the floor. Breathe in and out several times as you relax deeply. Inhale as you raise your head up slowly. Let your gaze move upward as you lift your chin and stretch your neck backward. Then let your chest rise, carefully arching your back as you gradually raise your upper body, one vertebra at a time. Do not cause pain, nor go farther than is comfortable. Be sensitive to any discomfort, and stop if you feel any pain. Just lift to where you can, without strain. Use your back muscles rather than your arm muscles to help you rise up. Try to keep your trunk, legs, and feet on the floor. When you get to the top, hold the position as you breathe easily, in and out (Figure 10-5). Then exhale while reversing your motions, lowering yourself down slowly and carefully, relaxing your back one vertebra at a time. Finally, turn over and let your back rest completely flat on the floor.

Half-Locust, Ardha-Salabhasana, and Full Locust, Salabhasana

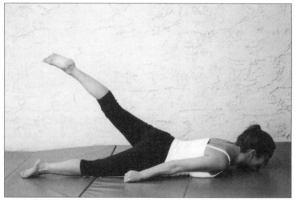

Figure 10-6: Half-locust

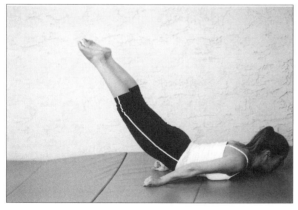

Figure 10-7: Full locust

The cobra pose begins at the upper part of the body and works downward. The locust pose begins at the lower half of the body and moves upward. Because of this opposite action, these two exercises are often done one after the other in routines, with the locust usually following the cobra.

The locust pose not only strengthens the back, trunk, and abdomen, but also firms the legs.

You can ease into the locust with the half-locust, raising one leg at a time. Begin by lying on your stomach with your arms extended down at your sides. Hold your hands in the form of fists, with thumbs facing toward your body, and rest the front of your chin (not the point) on the floor. Slowly raise your left leg as high as you can with comfort, leaving the other leg on the floor, as you inhale. Also keep your upper body and chin on the floor (Figure 10-6). Press down with your fists, especially on the left side. Hold and breathe normally, for several seconds, and then exhale as you slowly lower your leg. Repeat with the other leg.

For the full locust, lie in the same position as the half-locust, on your stomach with your arms at your sides and hands in fists. Push against the floor with your fists as you raise both legs up as far as you can, while inhaling (Figure 10-7). At first you will probably only raise your legs a few inches above the ground, but even this small distance can be beneficial. Hold the position as you breathe in and out for a few seconds, and then lower your legs slowly. Try to keep control of the movement. Do not attempt an extreme extension. Gradually over time the height will increase.

Fish Pose, Uttana Padasana

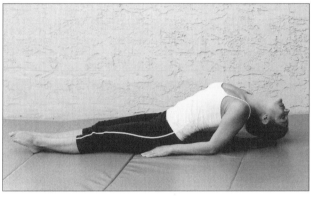

Figure 10-8: Fish pose

The fish pose offers an arching stretch to the shoulders, neck, and back. It is usually practiced after some of the inverted postures such as the shoulder stand or plough, because it exercises and stretches these areas in the opposite direction. The fish pose also can relieve stiffness in the neck, shoulders, and chest.

Lie flat on your back with your legs straight and feet together. Place your open hands flat on the floor, palms down, just under your thighs, thereby raising your lower body slightly off the ground. Breathe comfortably for a few moments and then inhale as you press down and in with your elbows, arch your back with care, and rest the top of your head on the floor (Figure 10-8). Pay attention to your back and do not cause pain. Breathe in and out as you try to relax more deeply, keeping your torso relaxed as well. When you feel ready, gently lift your head and drop your chin as you lower your body back down.

Inverted Asanas

Yoga is famous for its inverted postures. All systems of the body can benefit from being upside down, giving a brief relief from the usual downward pull of

> Inverted asanas promote health in many ways but they do have risks for people with certain health problems. So be sure to consult your doctor if you have any health conditions. Also listen to your own reactions and stop doing any inverted pose that causes discomfort or strain.

gravity. Yoga literature claims that inverted postures rest the heart and aid circulation. Practitioners also believe that being upside down improves mental functioning and adds vitality. According to yoga theory, a fresh supply of oxygen-rich blood is sent to the head, in these postures, giving the brain positive nourishment (Lidell and Narayani 1983; Smith 1986, pp. 134–35).

Even with all the potential advantages, you should exercise caution with inverted postures. Check with your doctor before you engage in these positions. There may be a risk for people with high blood pressure, heart problems, or a disk problem. You also should be careful of your neck and vertebrae, since these positions put pressure on these areas. And take care to perform them in the correct order, matched with poses that relax the areas affected, to counteract the pressure (see part 4). If you have any uncertainties, check with someone expert in these postures.

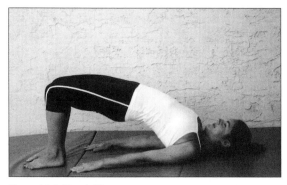

Figure 10-9: Easy bridge

Easy Bridge

Ease into inverted asanas by doing simpler, partially inverted asanas first. This position is a good introduction to inverted postures. It can be your substitute for the plow or shoulder stand if you have any physical problems or limitations that prevent you from doing inverted postures. The easy bridge can ease back pain and increase vitality.

Begin by lying on your back. Bend your knees and place your feet several inches apart, flat on the floor, bringing them up as close to your hips as you can. With your arms extended down toward your feet, palms facing down, raise your hips up and tuck your chin toward your chest. Your head, neck, and shoulders should remain relaxed, resting on the floor (Figure 10-9). Align your whole body in position. Hold for several seconds as you breathe in and out

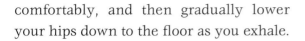

comfortably, and then gradually lower your hips down to the floor as you exhale.

Leg Raises, Preparation for the Plow and the Shoulder Stand

Yoga is a gradual process by which certain postures help to build the strength, flexibility, and balance needed for more difficult postures. The leg raise positions

You can ease into many yoga asanas by using aids, such as walls, blocks, balls, and cushions. The shoulder stand is a good example, where a wall can help you to gradually find your balance in the pose.

will prepare you for the classic inverted postures, such as the plow and the shoulder stand. Leg raises will help to gently strengthen your lower abdomen and thighs, and trim the waist.

Begin lying on your back in savasana. Bring your legs together and your arms in next to your sides. Raise your left leg up slowly as you exhale. Strive to keep the other leg and your whole back flat on the floor. Let your neck and shoulders remain relaxed. As you get stronger, this will become easier to do. Bring the leg up as high as you can without overly bending your knee. Hold for a few breaths in and out. Then inhale as you let your leg slowly return to the original position. Now raise and lower your right leg in the same way.

For the second phase of this exercise, slowly raise both legs together as you exhale. Only go as high as you can without bending your knees. Hold your legs in the air for several breaths in and out, and then slowly lower them back to the ground. To add difficulty to this exercise, pause briefly at 60 degrees, 45 degrees, 30 degrees, and 15 degrees as you lower your legs.

Shoulder Stand, Sarvangasana

The shoulder stand brings the many benefits of inverted postures. The increased circulation to the upper body not only helps to stimulate the mind, it also helps eliminate fatigue. The shoulder stand can relieve all the internal organs of their usual pull from gravity. Remember not to attempt this posture if you have any problems with your heart, blood pressure, or disks. Instead substitute the easy bridge whenever the shoulder stand appears in a routine.

You can start with a beginner's version of the shoulder stand that uses a wall as an aid. Begin by lying on your back close to an empty wall, with your legs up. Let them gently rest with your feet flat on the wall. Your knees will be bent. Gradually walk your feet up the wall as you lift your hips up as in the easy

Inverted postures can be very helpful in relieving foot strain. These asanas can help decrease swelling and fatigue in the feet after a long day of standing. You can even do a modified inversion by lying down close to a wall and resting your legs up against the wall. This is an easy way to give your feet a rest without straining. Hold this position for five minutes, breathing naturally as you relax.

bridge, and allow your head to rest on the floor, chin tucked in toward your chest. Place your elbows flat on the floor and let your hands support your back. Hold this position as you breathe comfortably in and out. When you feel ready, lower your legs and hips back to the floor and relax.

For the full version of the shoulder stand, begin with your arms extended at your sides with your palms flat on the floor. Draw your knees up as you did in the knee squeeze posture. Roll forward and back for a moment as you breathe, to allow your back to relax. When you feel ready, roll your legs backward, allowing your knees to rest on your forehead as you support your back with your hands, elbows resting on the ground. Then exhale as you smoothly raise your legs with control, straight up overhead until your body is in a nearly vertical position up to the shoulders (Figure 10-10). Try to keep your chest open and breathe. Maintain this position for thirty seconds or so, keeping your breathing easy and natural. With practice you can increase the time spent in shoulder stand. One of the difficulties in shoulder stand is getting your body straight and aligned.

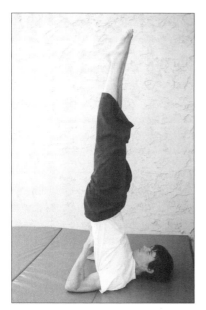

Figure 10-10: Shoulder stand

You may be able to make adjustments once you have found your balance. Make sure your two arms are aligned and that your palms are placed symmetrically to support your back. When you are correctly aligned with gravity, you should not have to strain to stay in position. If you feel a pull one way or the other, you are probably misaligned. Let your muscles relax in the position, and you will feel any tensions you may have begin to ease.

The neck is a vulnerable area and must be protected. The shoulder stand should be performed cautiously, with safety in mind. Beginners may want to add a folded blanket under the shoulders to give the neck some space. Work carefully with this asana, never pushing yourself into a painful position. If you find the shoulder stand uncomfortable, continue to do the beginner versions until you are stronger.

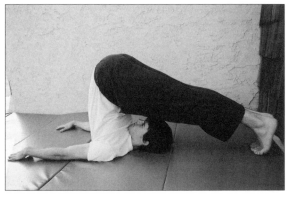

Figure 10-11: Plow

Plow, Halasana

The plow stretches the entire back side of the body. It also helps to enhance mental energy and induce calm. Often, one side of the neck and back muscles is tighter than the other. The plow helps to stretch the two sides equally to bring about balance.

The plow, like the shoulder stand, should be done with caution. Don't perform the plow if you have problems with your neck or back. Begin from the shoulder stand (Figure 10-10). Bring your knees down until they touch your forehead. Then slowly straighten your legs over your head, moving your toes toward the floor. The final position is for your toes to touch the floor, but only go as far as you can while remaining comfortable. You can do a modified plow by placing a pile of cushions close enough so that you can lower your legs to rest on them. You can also try lowering your legs and feet to rest on a wall behind you for support. You can spread and bend your knees or roll out of the pose if you need to.

Once your legs are extended, let your arms stretch out behind you, palms resting on the floor (Figure 10-11). If you do not feel balanced enough, keep your arms supporting your back as you did in the shoulder stand. Breathe comfortably, in and out. When you feel ready, bring your knees back in, to rest on your forehead, and then roll forward to a seated position.

Practice the asanas in this chapter to become familiar with what they are and how to do them. Then, when you perform them as part of your routine, you will be able to flow naturally from one posture to the next. Be gentle and gradual to allow your body to naturally become stronger and more flexible.

The posture becomes perfect when the effort of achieving it vanishes.
—Yogabhashya

THE ULTIMATE GOAL of practicing yoga postures is to be able to perform them effortlessly. At first, effort is needed to go into the pose. In time, the pose becomes easier, as muscles become relaxed and toned. Then one day a moment of absolute and complete comfort in the posture just happens. With patience and persistence, these moments extend, bringing greater calm and peace. This is the yoga experience of highly accomplished yogis.

A common stereotype of a yoga posture is to be seated cross-legged on the floor in an upright position. This is partly true, deriving from a tradition in India, where people often sat on the floor just as part of their daily routines. Today we are more accustomed to sitting in chairs, and so some people might feel intimidated by having to sit on the floor to do yoga. Fortunately, you do not have to be barred from practicing yoga if you are not able to sit comfortably cross-legged on the floor. Many of the sitting postures can be adapted to chair sitting, as long as you position your body correctly. Some of these adaptations are given at the end of this chapter. You may think of others.

Your Yoga Seat

Yoga offers a number of ways to sit on the floor. From these positions, different sitting asanas can be done. The important seat positions are shown here. Use the one that feels most comfortable to you to start, probably with an easy pose. As you become more flexible, you will be able to do the more advanced ones, leading to the classic lotus.

Discovering your "yoga seat" means to be able to sit effortlessly, freeing you for more meditation pursuits. Begin this process by becoming aware of sitting. Next time you are outdoors sit down on the ground. Close your eyes and place your hands palm down. Can you sense the support you get from the earth? Sit quietly and notice all the qualities of your experience.

Beginners who decide to sit on the floor will find it easier to use a firm cushion that will raise the hips three to six inches. This takes strain off the lower back and makes floor-sitting more comfortable. Eventually you may choose to sit without a pillow.

You should feel comfortable with your posture for sitting. If you are bothered by the sitting position, you may lose your concentration. Since concentration is a key to making progress in yoga, take some time to find the most comfortable sitting position. As you become more flexible, more positions will become easier to do.

Sitting Asanas

Prana energy flows around within the body, leaving through the hands and the feet. When you are seated cross-legged, energy can flow in a circle, continually nourishing the body rather than escaping. Thus, many traditional yoga sitting positions have the legs crossed in various ways.

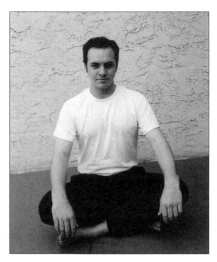

Figure 11-1: Easy pose

Easy Pose, Sukhasana

One of the easiest sitting positions is called the easy pose. The easy pose is very similar to the cross-legged position you may have used as a child when sitting on the floor.

Draw your left foot in until the heel is as far under your right thigh as possible without forcing. Then draw the right foot under the left thigh in the same way. Let your hands rest over your knees. Your legs will be crossed at the ankles. Most important is that you keep your spine, neck, and head balanced and held upright (Figure 11-1). This

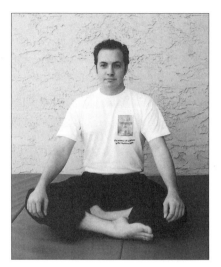

Figure 11-2: Auspicious pose

pose should be easy and natural to maintain over an extended period of time.

Auspicious Pose, Svastikasana

The auspicious pose is a slight variation of the easy pose. Bend your right leg and bring your right foot next to your left thigh. Then bend your left leg and bring your left foot up to your right thigh. Keep your spine, neck, and head aligned, balanced, and upright but not held rigid. This is another position that is easy to maintain for a long time (Figure 11-2).

Hero Pose, Virasana

The hero pose begins as in the easy pose, with your legs out in front of you. Draw the right foot in and turn the sole of your foot up. Take your left foot and place it over your right shin (Figure 11-3). Alternate which leg is under and which leg is over during different sessions. As in all sitting positions, keep your back straight and aligned, with neck and head balanced and upright, without excess tension. This position can serve as a practice for the next pose, the lotus position. In fact, this position is sometimes called the half-lotus.

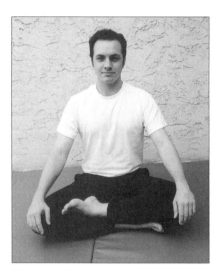

Figure 11-3: Hero pose

Experiment with the different sitting positions to find which one feels most comfortable for you. As you do yoga regularly, you may find that more sitting asanas become possible for you. Keep in mind that being able to relax as you sit will allow you to stay focused and aware. So try to find a sitting position that lets you be at ease.

Even though the lotus is the classic yoga sitting position, don't lose sight of the true meaning of sitting. Ultimately, the yoga seat should be effortless, completely still, allowing you to feel your Oneness with the universe. Straining to keep your body in an uncomfortable position that you are not ready to do will only detract from your inner transformation.

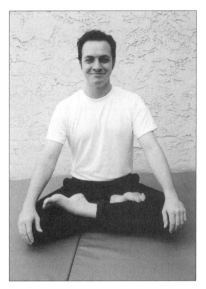

Figure 11-4: Lotus pose

Lotus Pose, Padmasana

The lotus pose is an ancient position described in the *Hatha Yoga Pradipika*. Some people find that they can do the lotus position without effort. Other people find it difficult because of their body type or level of flexibility. Keep in mind that comfort is always important, so don't try to force your body into this position if it does not feel good.

To perform the lotus position (Figure 11-4), place your right foot on the left thigh, and your left foot on the right thigh. Your legs are locked, making it easy to maintain the position over time (as long as the position is comfortable). Let your hands rest on your knees. You can touch your thumb to your index finger, forming a circle.

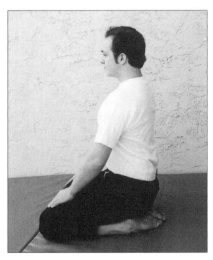

Figure 11-5: Pelvic pose

Pelvic Pose, Vajrasana

The pelvic pose is a kneeling position. Kneel on the floor and then sit back on your heels, keeping your back upright (Figure 11-5). To be more comfortable, place a small cushion under the backs of your legs or shins, to sit on. Some people may prefer this position to cross-legged ones, while others may have the opposite reaction. Let your body be your guide as to how to sit most comfortably.

Variation

If you find that you are unable to sit comfortably in any of the traditional positions, try some alternatives. You can use a straight-backed chair with a small pillow placed behind your lower back. You may be able to sit on a small pillow on the floor with your back against a wall and legs stretched out in front of you. Experiment to find what works best for you.

Active Sitting Asanas

The sitting postures included here will be used as part of the yoga routines described in part 4. Read the instructions carefully and practice the positions to get to know them. This will help you to be able to flow smoothly from one posture to the next when performing your yoga routine.

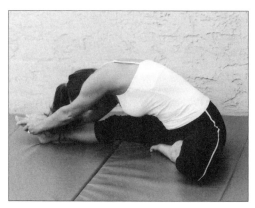

Figure 11-6: Alternate leg stretch

Alternate Leg Stretch, Udhitta Padasana

The alternate leg stretch is a good beginner stretch, because anyone can do it to some degree. This position will relax and stretch the back, neck, trunk, and abdomen. It will also help to tone these areas.

Begin as if you are going to sit in the auspicious pose, by tucking your left heel as close to your right thigh as is comfortable. Let your right leg extend out straight sideways. Raise both arms straight up overhead and inhale. Then gently move forward over the extended leg as you bring your hands down to your leg and exhale. Continue forward as far as you can, letting your hands slide down to hook around your foot, if possible (Figure 11-6). At the same time, let your neck muscles relax as you lower your head. If you can reach the full stretch of this posture, your head will rest on your leg, but most beginners will only get partway down. Remember not to push beyond what is comfortable. Hold the position as you breathe in and out several times, and then slowly and smoothly sit back up as you inhale. Switch your feet and repeat the exercise on the other side.

Stick Pose, Dandasana

Begin by lying down on your back with your feet together and hands next to your body, palms down on the floor. Inhale completely and then sit up slowly

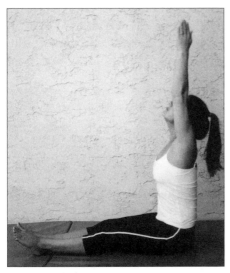

Figure 11-7: Posterior stretch pose, first part

with your legs remaining extended and palms on the floor, as you exhale. Come to an upright sitting position with your legs together, straight out in front of you, back straight, and head upright, palms down at your sides.

Try to keep the motion smooth. Work toward being able to lift yourself without support from your elbows. This position will help you to gain control over your abdominal muscles because of the tensing and relaxing required.

Posterior Stretch Pose, Paschimatanasana

From the upright position of the stick pose, raise your hands above your head, inhale completely (Figure 11-7), and then slowly bring your hands down near your toes as you bend forward, gently contracting your abdomen as you exhale (Figure 11-8). If you have enough flexibility, form a ring with your thumb and index finger and circle your big toe on each foot. Otherwise, hold your ankles or

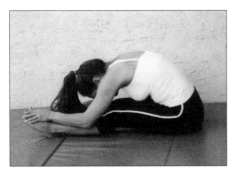

Figure 11-8: Posterior stretch pose, second part

legs. Make sure that you keep your back relatively straight as you bend forward. Don't round over from the middle of your spine in order to reach your toes. Maintain this position at the bottom of your exhale for a few seconds.

> ### Variation
>
> You can modify the posterior stretch pose if you find you are unable to sit comfortably on the floor with your legs extended straight out. To give yourself a gentler stretch, allow your knees to bend slightly as you bend forward. In time you will be able to perform the stretch with your legs straight.

Keep your knees relatively straight, and do not jerk or pull. If you feel that you need to raise your knees, you have bent too far. Just go as far as you can while keeping your legs straight. Breathe in and out for several breaths while you hold the position, relaxing a little more with each breath. When ready, gently straighten as you inhale. A variation for those with tight hamstrings is to bend the legs slightly at the knees, and do the forward bend as described above.

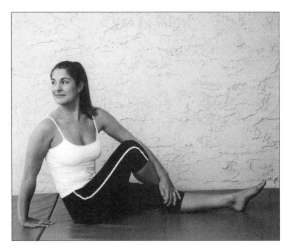

Figure 11-9: Twist pose

Twist Pose, Vakrasana

Twisting to the left and right will help you to add another dimension to your flexibility. The spinal twist pose tones the spinal column and ligaments, and improves digestion. Remember not to push beyond what is comfortable. There are many twisting variations in yoga that position the arms and legs in different ways, but this one is a good beginning twist.

Begin in the upright stick pose and raise your right knee, placing your foot flat on the floor on the outside of your straight left knee, and inhale completely. Place your right hand palm-down behind you, then cross your left arm over your raised right knee and grasp the outside of your straight knee. Gently twist your trunk to the right and look behind you as far as possible as you exhale completely. Keep your trunk area as straight as you can without forcing, and let your elbows remain relatively straight. Breathe in and out for several breaths as you hold the position, staying in alignment (Figure 11-9). Slowly switch to the other side, repeat the gentle twist, and hold in position, coordinating the movements with your breathing. Then return to center.

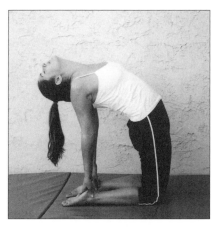

Figure 11-10: Camel pose

M any ancient cultures believed that all of nature had a spiritual quality. Not just animals, but also inanimate objects, such as rocks, trees, and mountains, were thought to be filled with spirit. People can feel their affinity with the universe and partake of the spirituality that is everywhere. Yoga carries on this tradition through asanas drawn from all forms of nature.

Camel Pose, Ustrasana

Many of the asanas in yoga have the names of animals and other natural things, such as the tree pose and the sun pose. These names have significance beyond the resemblance to natural forms. On a meditative level, the practice of yoga helps you to feel your oneness with the universe. By taking on the position of a camel or a cat, for example, you are also trying to get in tune with the spirit of this animal, to unify with it. Think about the spirit the posture could represent, and try to integrate that into your posture.

The camel pose is done from your knees. This position helps to limber the neck, back, thighs, and knees.

Kneel on a mat with your knees slightly separated. Begin to perform this posture by doing one side at a time. Bend back and take hold of your left heel with your left hand. Try to minimize the twist. Push your hips forward slightly. Breathe comfortably, relaxing as much as possible. Then, let go of your heel and straighten. Next, repeat the same position on your right side, grasping your right heel with your right hand. Practice balancing while leaning back.

When you feel ready, perhaps after some weeks of practice have passed, try both sides at the same time (Figure 11-10). Bend back and grasp your left heel with your left hand, and then grasp the right heel with the right hand. Push your hips forward as much as possible, and allow your head to relax backward. As you become even more comfortable and balanced with the pose, lift your chin slowly so that your head leans back. This is the complete camel pose. Hold for several seconds as you breathe normally. Then straighten as you sit up and remove your hands from your heels.

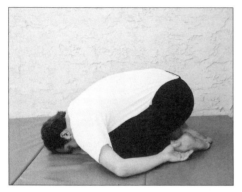

Figure 11-11: Child pose

Child Pose

The child pose is a good relaxing posture to perform after stretching by arching the back. It is easy to do. With practice you will be able to relax very deeply in this posture and will find it very refreshing. The child pose helps to relax and limber the shoulders, neck, and upper and lower back.

Sit on your feet in the pelvic pose, kneeling position. Bend forward slowly until your head touches the floor. Allow your arms to rest comfortably at your sides, with your elbows bent so that they can rest on the floor. You may need to shift and move slightly to find the most comfortable position. Breathe easily, and hold the position for a minute or so (Figure 11-11).

 Have you ever seen how completely relaxed an infant or young child is when sleeping? We all had this ability when we were young. The child pose can awaken in you your forgotten capacity to be absolutely relaxed.

If you cannot get comfortable, try reducing the angle a bit by folding your arms and placing your head on your arms. Do not hold the posture for longer than a second or two if you cannot feel at ease with it. Eventually, you will be able to enjoy this restful position, but it may take time.

Cat's Breath

Have you ever watched a cat stretch after a long nap? You will notice how he arches with his whole being, first one way and then the other. The cat's breath pose partakes of this spirit in cats to help you learn how to coordinate breathing with movement, while limbering your lower and middle back. Your abdomen will also get a workout.

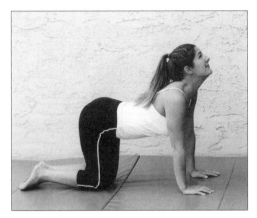

Figure 11-12: Cat's breath, first part

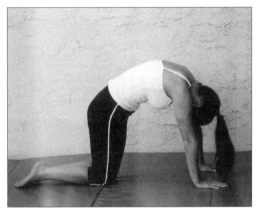

Figure 11-13: Cat's breath, second part

Begin on your hands and knees. Inhale as you arch your back with control and raise your head to look straight upward (see Figure 11-12). You should feel a full stretch along your entire back. Exhale, then smoothly and gently round your back as you pull your stomach in while tucking your chin down (see Figure 11-13). Repeat the entire sequence several times, moving and breathing slowly.

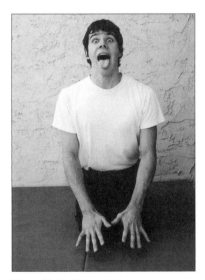

Figure 11-14: Lion pose

Lion Pose, Simhasana

The ferocity of the lion is unparalleled in nature. You can invigorate yourself by drawing upon the fierce side of your own nature. Unlike some of the slow, gradual poses, the lion pose can be performed with intensity. This exercise helps to tone your facial muscles and release emotional tension. Following the exercise, relax the face and neck areas.

The lion is performed kneeling. Place your hands on your knees and inhale completely. Then exhale sharply as you lean forward. At the same time, tense and separate your fingers, tense the muscles in your face and neck, open your eyes wide as you open your mouth, stick out your tongue, and push it down toward your chin (see Figure 11-14). Hold for approximately fifteen seconds and then slowly withdraw your tongue, relaxing your eyes, face, and neck, as well as your fingers, as you settle back into a kneeling position.

The lion has been a symbol of many admirable qualities, such as strength, alertness, leadership, and intensity. When performing the lion pose, imagine your energy rising. You are intensely aware and highly alert, ready to meet your life with self-confidence.

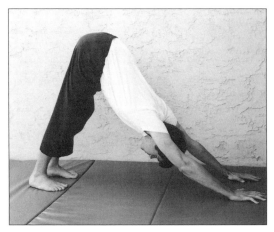

Figure 11-15: Dog pose

Dog Pose

The dog pose is part of the sun salutation series that is presented in part 4. It stretches and releases tension throughout the entire back of the upper body.

The dog pose is first performed from a kneeling position. Begin on your knees with your hands down on the floor in front of you, in a position similar to the way a dog stands. Breathe comfortably and relax. Then, inhale as you go up on the balls of your feet and raise your hips high in the air, while bending forward. Lower your head down toward the floor and straighten your arms, with fingers spread on the floor. Your entire back will stretch naturally from this position. Hold as you breathe, trying to relax. Stretch a little more if you can do so without discomfort by pushing your heels down flat on the floor (Figure 11-15). Then, exhale as you slowly return to the kneeling starting position.

Yoga Mudra Pose

This posture has been called the symbol of yoga representing unity, because the whole body makes a continuous circle. When you sit in this position, you can feel a sense of oneness throughout your body, as your head feels unified with your legs, your arms unified with your back, and so forth. Notice what interrelationships you sense for yourself.

This posture is believed to tone the internal

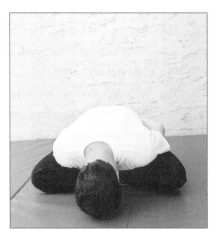

Figure 11-16: Yoga mudra pose

organs and calm the nerves. It also helps to enhance vitality and latent energies. You may experience serenity and calm as well.

To perform the yoga mudra, sit in the most comfortable cross-legged position. Naturally flexible people can use the lotus position, but the easy pose will also be effective. Place your hands behind your back, wrapping your right hand around your left. Inhale and then bring your forehead down toward the ground by bending forward smoothly from the trunk (Figure 11-16). Maintain the posture for several breaths, and then bring your hands back around to the front and let them rest on your legs. Return to an erect sitting position, and inhale.

Try sitting on the floor at times during the day to get used to it. Practice the sitting asanas to familiarize yourself with each one. These positions will become part of your yoga routine.

Mudras are a traditional form of symbolic gestures used along with meditation to bring about higher consciousness. Yoga and Tibetan Buddhism make the most extensive use of mudras, but they are also found in other meditative disciplines. When performing a mudra such as the yoga mudra, you place the body in a certain position and then meditate on the symbolic meaning. For the yoga mudra, a topic for meditation is Oneness and unity.

From a Chair

You can modify most of these positions for sitting in a chair. Choose a stable, four-legged chair to use, or a sturdy living-room chair. Make sure the area around it is clear and safe. A mirror on the wall can give you feedback. When performing a yoga pose sitting in a chair, keep your spine, neck, and head upright, just as in the floor-sitting positions. Make sure your thighs are parallel to the floor, and your lower legs perpendicular to the floor. If the chair is too high to do this, you may need to place a book or pillow under your feet on the floor to raise them up. Let your hands rest on your knees, with your arms away from your ribcage. Be careful with your balance when you are leaning over. Try bending forward carefully over one knee and then the other as you lightly hold your leg. You can do a partial forward bend as well, keeping your legs together. Upright twists can also work well. But use caution. Hold on to the back of the chair for extra support. Remember to keep your spine straight as you twist. As usual, do not use force. Be gentle. Experiment carefully with the different positions, always coordinating them with breathing and focused attention, and you will find that your flexibility and strength can improve. Be creative with your methods. The important thing is to actually perform yoga, not just to force yourself into the poses in traditional ways. In time, your flexibility will improve.

You can perform yoga sitting in a chair at work, in a seat on an airplane, or in other unusual situations where you may want to do a bit of yoga to relax and loosen up. Experiment with some of the twists, forward bends, and leg raises. Remember to move slowly, to coordinate your breathing, and to keep your attention fully focused on what you are doing.

breathing:
pranayama

*Pranayama is the conscious, deliberate regulation
of the breath replacing unconscious patterns of breathing. . . .
The regular practice of pranayama reduces the obstacles
that inhibit clear perception.*
—The Yoga Sutras of Patanjali

As ONE OF the eight limbs of yoga, breathing has a primary place in yoga practice. Although people breathe without any deliberate thought or effort, the deliberate breathing practices of yoga can have a positive effect on both the mind and body. Breathing is a bridge that closely links mind and body together. For example, when we are excited, our breathing becomes more rapid and our thoughts race; when relaxed, breathing slows and the mind becomes calm. Those who use breathing techniques have more control over themselves and their emotional reactions.

These breathing exercises are called pranayama. The word *prana* means "vitality" and "flowing within." Prana is the life force that permeates everything. Similar to the Chinese concept of *chi*, prana is somewhat like a form of energy that flows throughout the universe. Each person has a flow of prana that can be raised, lowered, and directed.

Ayama signifies "to stretch or extend." Thus the term "pranayama" means a way to extend the flow of vitality within. Through deliberate modifications and methods, pranayama brings breathing under conscious control. Consciousness can direct the flow of prana into and out of the body. Yogis believe that when we get excited or upset, prana tends to leave the body. But through pranayama breathing exercises, we can bring prana back into the body, thereby revitalizing it.

"Pranayama really means controlling the motion of the lungs, and this motion is associated with the breath. . . . Prana is not breathing, but controlling that muscular power which moves the lungs. . . . When this prana has become controlled, then we shall immediately find that all the other actions of prana in the body will slowly come under control." (Nikhilananda 1953, p. 595)

For thousands of years, breathing has been a focus of meditation to raise energy, relax, and get a deeper glimpse into the inner being. Taoism, Zen, and yoga all consider breathing the gateway to higher consciousness.

Anatomy of the Breath

Yoga practitioners have analyzed breathing in order to develop its use to the fullest potential. Breathing can be divided into four parts. First is the inhalation, *puraka*, when the air is brought into the body. Next comes held-in-breath, *kumbhaka*, a moment between breathing in and out. Exhalation, *rechaka*, lets the air out, followed by a pause, or the held-out-breath, *shunyaka*, before the pattern repeats again.

After years of disciplined pranayama practice, skillful yogis can vary their rhythms and processes of breathing at will. The process starts with gradual, gentle changes to normal breathing and builds from there. By changing the pattern, timing, and force of different parts of the cycle of breathing, practitioners can gain control over processes that usually seem to be automatic.

Begin with Awareness

Breathing is usually an unconscious process that takes care of itself. But yogis believe that when we leave the breathing process to chance, we use only a small portion of our potential for self-control and health, resulting in poor habits of tension and restriction. Awareness can help you to gently redirect your breathing and develop new and better breathing habits, which will bring about greater vitality, calm, and deeper relaxation. The first step in pranayama is conscious awareness. So begin by turning your attention to breathing.

Control of breathing must always be done carefully and gradually. Ultimately, the breath happens of itself naturally. You just help it along. The art of yoga lies in being able to deliberately enhance the natural potentials of the body. With corrective techniques you can bring about the best possible functioning. Your body will respond to gentle, gradual extension of its capacities without forcing anything.

Join your thinking with your senses to help you attune to breathing. One time-honored method is counting. The other is listening. Experiment with both of these exercises to see which seems more natural to you. Concentration in yoga begins as an inner experience. Either exercise can teach you to concentrate on breathing, an important stepping-stone to successful yoga practice. The two exercises that follow will help you to develop your powers of concentration.

If you are new to meditation and to yoga, try doing each of these exercises for a brief time. Set a timer for one minute and then begin. As you become comfortable with doing them for a short time, you will be able to increase the duration of your concentration for longer periods of time. Don't force it, but be persistent. You will be pleasantly surprised at how your powers of concentration can be developed with practice.

> In yoga breathing exercises, try to keep your breathing as natural and comfortable as possible. Don't take overly deep breaths or breathe too quickly. You may, at times, try to lengthen or shorten a breath, but do it gently, gradually, and carefully. In time, your breath control improves.

Focus on Breathing: Counting the Breaths

This ancient yoga exercise can help you learn to keep your attention on breathing. Sit cross-legged on a pillow on the floor, or on a chair if you find sitting on the floor uncomfortable. (See chapter 11 for instructions on sitting positions.) Close your eyes and begin inwardly counting each breath. Consider the entire breath: first inhale and then exhale as one breath. Count up to ten and then begin again. If your concentration wanders away from the count, gently bring it back as soon as you notice. Over time, you will be able to stay focused on your breathing at will.

Focus on Breathing: Listening to Breathing

Some people find that listening to breathing comes easier than counting the breaths. Sit comfortably and close your eyes. Pay close attention to the sound

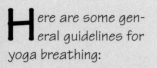

Here are some general guidelines for yoga breathing:

☞ Always breathe through your nose.

☞ Keep your posture upright to allow the free flow of air.

☞ If you ever start to feel dizzy during a breathing exercise, stop doing the exercise and breathe normally.

of the air as it enters your nose. Keep your attention focused on the sound as it exits again. Continue focusing attention on the sound of breathing for a few minutes. If you get distracted, gently bring your attention back to the sound of your breathing.

You can hear your breathing more easily by placing your hands lightly over your ears. Notice how the sound is amplified. After you have done this for a short time you will become sensitized to your breathing sounds, making it easier to stay attuned.

The Complete Breath

The complete breath is one of the cornerstones of yoga, used along with most of the postures to help you get the most out of your practice of yoga. It can be performed standing up, lying down, or sitting. A complete breath naturally brings about movement of the chest, ribcage, diaphragm, and abdomen. When done correctly, the complete breath fills the lungs, expanding them forward, sideways, and backward.

Without realizing it, people often get into the poor habit of holding their chest, ribcage, diaphragm, and abdomen rigid while breathing. Such inflexibility prevents a full breath from happening. As a result, energy becomes blocked or stuck, resulting in discomfort and even illness. The complete breath is the first step in a process to free breathing as it frees the body. The complete breath takes full advantage of all the muscles used in breathing. By practicing the complete breath, you learn to let go of unnecessary tensions, releasing your energy to flow naturally and fully.

To begin the complete breath, stand with your feet together and hands down at your sides, palms facing in toward your body. Let your head sag forward slightly, and exhale. Slowly begin inhaling as you raise your head up and arms out from your sides, arms straight with palms up. Let your lungs be completely filled with air when your hands meet up above your head. Hold for a moment and then slowly begin exhaling as you lower your arms. All your air should be expelled when your arms are back down at your sides.

The complete breath can also be done sitting up. Find a comfortable seated posture. Begin by inhaling. When you are first learning, place your hands on your upper abdomen to feel the motion as you breathe. Your hands should move out and your fingers should move slightly apart as your lungs fill with air. Exhale and let your abdomen deflate, bringing your fingers together again.

Expanding the abdomen is just part of the complete breath. The diaphragm, ribcage, and chest are also involved. Place your hands on your diaphragm/rib area to feel this part of the breath. As you inhale, notice how your diaphragm naturally expands downward as your ribs spread outward. Your chest also expands, and your shoulders rise slightly. The complete inhale, done correctly, will bring about movement in your abdomen, diaphragm, ribs, chest, and shoulders.

Exhaling is just the opposite. Begin by relaxing your chest first, then your ribcage, and finally lightly tighten your stomach muscles to help push the last bit of air out. Your chest and ribcage contract, and your shoulders drop with exhalation. One complete inhale and exhale, with one following the other, make up a complete breath.

Inhalation and exhalation should be evenly timed, with a slight pause. You may want to count to four as you inhale and then to four as you exhale. You can breathe for up to six counts. Do what feels comfortable.

Beginners often find it easier to do a longer exhale, but you should spend the same amount of time inhaling and exhaling. This probably means shortening the exhale rather than lengthening the inhale. Feel this out for yourself. You should not feel as if you are forcing your breathing to be longer or shorter. Listen to your own inner rhythms.

Even though you are deliberately trying to breathe in a certain way, keep it as relaxed and natural as possible. Breathing should not be strained, hard, or sudden. As your breathing becomes more balanced and comfortable, you may feel more relaxed and calm as well.

Cleansing Breath One

Yoga philosophy encourages people to increase their flow of prana to help them revitalize. Certain breathing patterns have a cleansing effect by forcing out old, stale air. Then, clean, fresh air can bring prana in.

One exercise used to achieve this is to alter the rhythm of breathing, clearing out impurities and making room for clean, fresh air. You may like performing this exercise outdoors in fresh air—at the beach, in the woods, or in a garden, for example.

Sit comfortably and breathe consciously for a few moments, to center yourself in your breathing. When you feel ready, inhale for a count of three with a complete breath in. Then hold the air for a comfortable count of one or two. Exhale for four counts with a complete breath out, and hold for one or two counts. Practice this gently and softly, making your breathing as relaxed as possible. Over time, you may be able to increase the length of each part of the breath, but keep the ratios the same. Controlling the timing of breathing is a more advanced skill that develops very slowly with practice. Be patient, because these skills take time to master.

Cleansing Breath Two

This exercise uses the abdominal area to push out stale air that can accumulate from shallow, incomplete breathing. Stand or sit upright and draw a full breath in. Then exhale through your nose with a quick, short burst as you pull your abdomen in. Your exhalation should make an audible sound from air pushing out. Work up to six or so repetitions, but don't push yourself. If you feel any discomfort or dizziness, stop doing this exercise and rest for a few minutes.

Alternate Nostril Breath

This exercise balances the energy currents on both sides of the body. It can also enhance concentration. Curl the first two fingers of your right hand, and rest your thumb against the curled fingers, pointing up. Extend your fourth and fifth fingers out straight. Cover your right nostril with your thumb and inhale through your left nostril, allowing the air to flow fully, as in the complete breath. Then shift your hand to block the left nostril with your extended fingers, and exhale through your right nostril, performing a complete exhale. Inhale fully through the right nostril, and then block it so that you can exhale with the other. Alternate back and forth in this way for five to ten breath cycles.

Advanced Breathing

When control of breathing is developed to a high level, advanced pranayama exercises are used. The advanced breathing techniques are not usually taught until the student has developed proficiency with the earlier pranayama exercises included in this book.

One of the more mystical practices of yoga is called kundalini. It uses breathing and meditation. Kundalini refers to cosmic energy. It is usually described metaphorically as a coiled snake lying dormant at the base of the spine. When the kundalini is awakened by regular practice of pranayama, meditation, and asanas, it moves up through the spine to the brain, like an electric current moving along a cable.

Yogis believe that people have several kinds of bodies coexisting in parallel with each other, such as the astral body and the subtle body. The practice of kundalini yoga activates these other bodies.

The kundalini passes through and pauses at a series of "stations" called chakras. The chakras are part of the astral body, but they correspond to parts of the physical body. For example, there is a chakra at the level of the solar plexus, another at the throat. Each chakra has specific purposes that can be activated by certain breathing and meditation practices. Prana is the link between them.

> Yoga can be practiced in many ways and at many levels. Some people look only for the health and fitness benefits. But those who delve into the mystical dimension can discover an expansion of consciousness. Kundalini breathing techniques are an exploration of the mystical side of yoga.

For example, *bhastrika*, one of the most powerful exercises, creates a bellows by pumping and then retaining breath in exacting ways. The *bhandas* are locks that regulate the flow of energy. The air is held in a definite place in the body, such as the throat or abdomen, by tightening appropriate muscles, and then released. These and other advanced practices help hold and direct energy up through the kundalini.

New levels of consciousness are experienced as the energy travels up through each chakra. These esoteric practices take a high development of yogic skills and should be undertaken only with careful guidance from an experienced guru.

Integrating Breathing with Postures

Careful use of the breath is always incorporated into the yoga postures. This exercise will help you begin integrating breathing patterns with movements, while also limbering your spine. If you can sit comfortably on your feet with your knees together in pelvic pose, vajrasana, do so, as this allows the spine more freedom. Otherwise, sit any way that is comfortable for you. Breathe in through your nose as you raise your ribcage and arch your back forward slightly, giving a gentle stretch to your spine. As you exhale, round your back slightly in the opposite direction and tuck your head forward. Repeat the gentle movements, coordinating them with your breathing, for three to five repetitions. Remember not to force the movements or the breathing. Keep both relaxed and gradual, and in time you will find that you become more limber as you grow accustomed to breathing with motion.

Integrating Yoga Breathing into Everyday Life

Specific breathing exercises are performed during yoga workouts. But it is also beneficial to turn your attention to breathing without exercising or imposing a fixed pattern. So take a few relaxed, aware breaths randomly throughout your day. You may also notice that there are times when you are unnecessarily holding your breath or forgetting to breathe. After you become aware of this, you may be able to gently let go and breathe normally. Be willing to take an inward glance here and there to develop better habits. Relaxed breathing optimizes energy for more vitality throughout the day.

meditation

*He who has faith, who is intent on it (knowledge)
and who has controlled his senses, obtains knowledge
and having obtained it, goes quickly to the highest peace.*
—Bhagavad-Gita

THE LAST FOUR LIMBS of yoga in Patanjali's system deal with mental development that leads to the highest spiritual attainment: peace and happiness. The fifth limb, pratyahara, is a transition point from the practice of asanas and pranayama, along with the yamas and niyamas, into meditation. The sixth limb is concentration, called dharana. Contemplation, dhyana, the seventh limb, comes next, leading to the subsequent experience of enlightened bliss, or samadhi, the eighth limb.

Meditation can have a profoundly positive effect on everyday life. Even meditating for just a few minutes of the day can set a process in motion that leads to deeper calm and fuller awareness.

Pratyahara

Pratyahara is the withdrawal of perception from the mere use of the senses. Yoga trains and disciplines the mind to learn to observe without the senses or subjective consciousness intervening, so that nothing interferes with direct perception. According to yoga philosophy, because the senses are turned outward toward the material world, they cannot be turned inward toward spiritual realities and higher consciousness. So, when the mind is withdrawn from the material world and disengaged from the senses, consciousness is freed for meditation.

We are accustomed to filling our perceptions with our sensory experience. We direct our attention to things, events, and people in the world. Pratyahara meditation shows us how to direct our awareness in a different way, leading to calm and clarity.

To understand pratyahara, consider its two sides: not-doing and doing. Withdrawing from distraction and unnecessary thought is the not-doing side of pratyahara. When we withdraw from involvement in outer, less important concerns, we conserve our energy and free our consciousness for positive use. Actively turning inward, focusing the light of consciousness toward concerns that matter, is the doing side of pratyahara. Then concentration, contemplation, and the consequent samadhi, the last three limbs, can take place. Mental abilities can be enhanced by following these processes.

Exercises in Pratyahara

Take a few minutes of the day when you can set aside the time for pratyahara. The classic yoga way to perform pratyahara is lying down in savasana pose. Remember, when lying down, that meditation is not sleep. Be aware.

The place you choose may be special, calm, peaceful, or somewhat quiet, where distractions are minimal. Turn up the temperature slightly or have a blanket handy if you think you might get cold, because your body temperature may drop a bit as you lie still. Pratyahara can be done in the morning, or late at night, or after work. It is also part of the meditation period at the end of a yoga workout. There is a natural rhythm for you. Trust that rhythm, and use it for beneficial purposes.

Lie quietly and relax. At first your thoughts may wander around, and little things will distract you. But be patient and you will be rewarded by a gradual quieting down of your thoughts.

Pratyahara Exercise: Narrowing the Field

Yoga will help you to become aware and let go of anything extra. People often carry extra tension without realizing it.

Turn your attention away from the outer world toward the inner, the experience of your body. Notice what sensations you have in each area. Begin at your head. Pay attention to your face or neck. How are you holding the muscles? Are you tightening them unnecessarily? If possible, relax any unnecessary tightness that you notice. Then direct your attention down toward your shoulders. Pay close attention to them. Mentally trace out how wide your shoulders are. Notice whether you are holding the muscles tight, and let go if possible. Continue down through your body, first paying close attention and then trying to relax any extra tension. You may be surprised to notice areas that are tightly tensed, but don't need to be. If your attention wanders away from your body to outer concerns, bring it back. But do not force yourself to relax. Simply notice where you can or cannot relax, and gently keep trying to increase the relaxation.

Pratyahara Exercise: Withdrawing the Senses

This exercise will help you narrow the focus away from too many thoughts at once. Calm awareness develops with practice.

Lie down in savasana pose. Withdraw your attention from outer surroundings as much as possible. So don't, for example, listen to the sound of traffic outside. Try to relax your thoughts just as you relaxed your body. Let go of any irrelevant thoughts, and simply stay with this peaceful, relaxed moment. You don't need to think about anything in particular. If your thoughts wander away, gently bring them back to this calm moment as soon as you can.

Dealing with Resistance to Pratyahara

If you have difficulty doing the pratyahara exercises, think about the habitual ways that you place your attention on the outer world. For example, are you always planning what you will do next, rehearsing in your mind? Do you have hidden assumptions that might be preventing you from relaxing now? Sometimes people believe they must be busy to be happy, and that relaxation is just laziness. Delve deeply and question these hidden assumptions. Everyone has individual ways, so don't judge or blame yourself, just observe. If you take a nonjudgmental attitude, your inner mind will open up to you as an ally.

Once you become aware of a habitual tendency, or an assumption that misdirects your attention, make a small change during your pratyahara practice. For example, if you notice yourself planning, thinking about what you will be doing after your pratyahara session, stop planning and bring your attention

Meditation is accessible to everyone, but some people may find it difficult to do at first. If you find that you can't do the exercises in this chapter, try shortening the time to just thirty seconds or even less. Sometimes people start with only a moment or two. In time you will be able to extend your meditation.

back to the moment. Or if you are recalling what you were doing earlier, or worrying about a problem, let go of the memories and worries, for now. Whenever you notice your thoughts not on your practice during pratyahara, gently bring them back, and eventually, distracting thinking will stop.

Concentration

The youth of the warrior class in India learned archery, to train their focus and acuity. One famous story about Arjuna's archery training describes a contest. Arjuna's class was instructed to draw their bows and aim for a bird perched in a distant tree, to see who was the best. While the students held their bows taut, the teacher asked, "What do you see?"

The first student answered, "I see a field, some trees, and a bird in one of the trees."

The second student said, "I only see the tree that has the bird in it."

Arjuna's response was, "All I see is the eye of the bird." The teacher declared Arjuna the winner!

Correct focus of attention is the beginning of concentration. Concentration is focused into a single point and kept there. This one-pointed, selective concentration can be learned through disciplined attention. Exercises that help train your concentration will prepare your mind for meditation. Deliberately cultivating perception and attention to outward objects and experiences help you gain control and permits you to turn your attention at will to inner concerns and experiences.

Attention is the key to unlocking the powers of the mind. Begin to train yourself to respond at will to whatever you choose to pay attention to. Simple concentration exercises are the starting point for learning meditation. In the yoga model of consciousness, your deliberate will and intention make a difference, so set your mind and try your best. Combined with commitment to the yamas and niyamas, concentration intensifies the experience of yoga. Then meditation on the experience permits the full effects to take place.

Patanjali's aphorisms, the *Yoga Sutras*, give structured guidelines to follow. In Patanjali's time, actual teaching of techniques was from guru to student, by word of mouth, not through books. Patanjali assumed that a guru would be instructing his readers in actual details. If you find that after study and practice over time you still cannot focus your attention, seek the help of an experienced yoga teacher.

One-pointed concentration is a classic meditation exercise that has been used through the ages to sharpen attention. The capacity to keep your attention focused at will has many useful applications in everyday life.

Activity for Concentration

Any basic activity or thing can be used as an object of concentration. Pick an object that you find interesting, such as a painting or sculpture you like. Place it in clear view. Sit upright in easy pose and look at the object. Keep your attention focused on it, and notice everything you can: color, texture, shape, size, function, and meaning, if relevant. Don't think about anything else. If your attention wanders away, bring it back to the object. Begin with just two or three minutes of concentration. Gradually increase the time, as you become able to maintain your focus. Skills in concentrating improve with practice.

Concentration on Sound

Concentration can be placed on a sound as well. In this exercise you focus attention on a sound and concentrate on it. It is best if the sound is simple, although there are groups of sounds and complex chants that may be learned over time.

The word *mantra* comes from the Sanskrit roots *manas*, "mind," and *tra*, "tool." Chanting a mantra is a way to focus attention and direct oneself into union with enlightened consciousness. Mantras don't have any "magic" of their own; they work through the mind that experiences them.

Listening to music is a form of concentration on sound. If you have ever found yourself lost in some music you like, you have experienced spontaneous concentration on sound. You can develop this ability deliberately by using the meditation exercises included here.

Om is a sound that is universal and known in many traditions. In yoga philosophy, om is a primary mantra: a sound that can be used to vibrate the body and activate energy centers, as well as clear the mind by listening. So mantra yoga is direct communication with the world and the body.

Begin with the sound, "ah," then say "oh," and then close your lips and finish with "mmm." Glide the sounds together as one combined syllable. Make the sound "om." As you do, focus all your attention on it: listen to it, feel the physical vibrations. Concentrate your attention only on the sound om. Do this for several minutes, increasing the duration, as you are able.

Concentration on Breathing: Following the Breath

Pranayama practices may be used for concentration. Focus all your attention on breathing as you do it, to develop the deep, one-pointed focus of attention of yogic concentration. This will also lead into deep meditation. In effect, these practices of yoga can all be used for concentration and meditation, using trained consciousness.

For this exercise, sit cross-legged on a pillow, sit on a chair, or lie down on the floor on your back. Most importantly, allow your breathing passages to be relatively relaxed. Close your eyes and turn your attention to your breathing. Breathe through your nose, not your mouth. Notice the air as it comes in through your nose, then flows down into your lungs and then out again. Pay close attention to how your chest, diaphragm, stomach, and back move as you breathe. Don't interfere with the natural pattern of breathing. Just relax and breathe normally, as you keep your attention focused on the process of breathing. If your attention wanders, gently bring it back to focus on breathing. For those who find this exercise difficult to do, return to one of the previous two exercises. These skills respond to practice, so be patient and keep trying.

Body Sensations Concentration

Extend your concentration meditation into everyday life. You can practice it walking, standing, and lying down. Scan your body to be aware of your arms,

legs, and body sensations as you go about everyday activities. Pay close attention to your breathing. Be sure to breathe naturally, neither more deeply, nor
more shallowly than usual. Sometimes, one forgets to breathe naturally, due
to intense concentration. Concentration on very basic body sensations while
observing breathing can be beneficial.

Contemplation

Yoga is the method of yoking the mind through meditation, of using focused
awareness and concentration. Meditation begins by fixing the mind upon an
idea, concept, image, sound, or the like, and holding the focus so that the
enlightenment process can take place. Training the intellect to hold a thought
in mind allows it to be available to other thoughts in a chain of linked ideas.
This is contemplation, another aspect of mental training in yoga. Contemplation is a great mental tool for learning.

Originally, the concepts of yoga practice were not filled with detail. The
intent was to communicate the unity of reality, not the parts of it. And contemplation is a way of giving an opportunity to the mind to experience that
unity, through thought.

In yoga philosophy, mental abilities are gained from focus. These abilities
come about through immersion in the greater, universal consciousness. When
the individual consciousness tunes in to the universal mind, it becomes
capable of broader intuitions, which make empathy possible. The material
world is real, although individual consciousness of it may vary. Perfected consciousness can know objects as they are. And action leaves no trace in consciousness when yogic detachment is practiced. Each moment of experience
is let go of, not held in consciousness.

This yogic view of reality assumes that forming concepts about an object
through the rational thought process produces a cascade of imaginary objects
and perceptions based on the illusions of the individual consciousness rather
than on an actual object. Conceptual thought leads to limited perception. But
concepts without thought lead beyond themselves. Concepts can be tools
when used in this way.

Contemplation of a Task

Any simple task you do can be a focus of contemplation. Begin by focusing
on something you do regularly, such as preparing a meal at home or a report

We take for granted that a good way to understand things is to form concepts and draw conclusions. Yoga contemplation uses a different way of thinking, which instead of drawing conclusions, permits enlightened understanding.

at work. Concentrate on the task as you do it. Then observe the subsequent flow of ideas about it. For example, consider related types of food for the meal, or related issues for the report. Keep returning to the task itself. Let your ideas flow freely without forming a concept or drawing any conclusions about the task or your actions. This is a discipline.

Contemplation Exercise with a Concept

This exercise brings your focus of concentration inwards. Pick an object of thought. It could be an animal, a person, a material object, or an idea. Whatever you choose becomes your point of concentration. Contemplate all thoughts about it, anything that is related to it. If you have thoughts unrelated to the object of your concentration, bring them back to it.

Remember not to force yourself to attend. Do not get angry at yourself or try to discipline yourself too fiercely. Tension and uncertainty about concentration and contemplation can be destructive. Just relax, be calm; do the best you can at this moment, without concern for alternatives of better or worse. Stay focused on the exercise process itself. This, in itself, is concentration.

Once you have chosen your topic to contemplate, write it on paper or make a small drawing or model of it. Think of something related to it, and then return to the central idea as focus. Then consider another idea, related to the first, and then return to center. The related idea could be used as a focus, too.

For example, concentrate for a moment on the word *yoga*. Then think of one of the side topics in this book, such as asanas. Consider what they are, then return to the central word *yoga*. Do not lose the link. Then think of another topic, such as breathing with pranayama. Again, return to the central word, yoga. Keep the back-and-forth flow of thought. Think of each linked concept. You may want to note your thoughts down. Then come the links for contemplation/meditation, the play of thoughts and ideas concerning the meanings and their relationships. Hold these in mind with concentration, as you contemplate each of the aspects of yoga.

From Contemplation to Meditation

Following Patanjali's eight limbs of yoga meditation training, which begins with withdrawing the senses, concentration, and then contemplation, readies the mind for deeper unity: the immersion and oneness of samadhi. So meditation begins with the natural consequence of concentration on what you do or think, and step by step, the process leads to the development of enlightened consciousness.

Experiment with contemplation on all kinds of topics. You may enjoy using your mind in this different way. Be flexible.

Immerse yourself in the process, permitting the whole to form, the unified pattern of interrelationship. Be one with the unified pattern. It is like shifting from two dimensions, on paper, to a bird's-eye, three-dimensional view, including and embracing all. This same process can be used with groups of concepts. Such meditation has no end to its usefulness. The state of samadhi follows contemplation. For a moment, you forget yourself in fascination and become part of something more. You have new thoughts, creative and fresh. From where they come, we do not know.

Samadhi is a unifying of the self with the wider spiritual nature. The distinction between subject and object melts away into a feeling of complete immersion in universal Oneness.

Meditation brings the higher consciousness referred to as samadhi, harmony with the deeper spiritual nature of the world. Be in harmony with yourself and the greater universe. Take seriously each moment in each posture. Breathe with awareness. Point the light of your awareness beyond your individual thoughts of each part, toward the greater whole. Yoga meditation can help you not only to get the most out of your practice sessions, but also to discover spiritual depth in everyday life.

Meditation with Visualization

Lie down in savasana pose, or sit up in one of the seated postures. Close your eyes and visualize a single point. Then, imagine that the point gets smaller and smaller, until it vanishes to nothingness. Stay in this moment of focused attention, just here and now, in effortless stillness, and become part of the whole.

This method of expanding consciousness can be applied in many useful ways. You can master your area of learning with this totally focused attention. So begin to apply your concentration to your positive goals.

Meditation does not have to be limited to your yoga practice. You can meditate at different times during the day. The extra practice will help to improve your skills. The benefits of meditation are far-reaching and satisfying. Greater calm, self-awareness, and a general feeling of well-being are only a few of the positive changes you will experience from the regular practice of meditation.

practice sequences

YOGA IS PRACTICED in a sequence of asana postures. The sequences have a well-planned order that makes the most of their benefits, while carefully safeguarding against injury. By performing a consistent sequence of movements over time, you are practicing yoga as it has been done through the ages.

Each of the sequences included in part 4 has a different emphasis. The first two series are a good place for the beginner to start. Later sequences will invigorate, strengthen, and add flexibility. You can combine several of the series, depending upon your goals.

The postures in each series are drawn from asanas taught in part 3, with some additional variations. The individual poses are described again briefly in part 4 so that you can move through the series without having to flip back through the book for descriptions. However, you may find it helpful at times to refer to the complete detailed descriptions given in part 3.

Begin by performing the routines dynamically, moving slowly from one

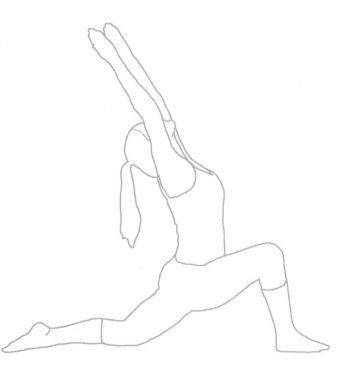

position to the next. As you improve in your skill, try to hold the positions longer. Static posing can be more challenging. Do not neglect your breathing while holding the postures. Keep it gentle and relaxed. As you inhale, let your abdomen expand, and as you exhale, let your abdomen contract. Eventually you will be able to hold a position without effort. This comes from gradual, gentle, consistent practice.

sun salutation: an invigorating morning routine

*Even the wise man acts in conformity
with his own nature. Beings follow nature.*
—Bhagavad-Gita

THE SUN GIVES AND sustains life, and for this, yogis feel gratitude. The sun salutation represents this gratitude as respect for the wonders of the universe of which we are a small, yet significant, part. Just as the sun gives its energy to the world, the sun salutation is believed to energize the entire body. The dynamic movements reach from head to toe.

One of the most important aids to the successful practice of yoga is to have a set sequence of asanas balanced with pranayama and meditation that you can do. Think about what you are hoping to gain, for example, becoming more invigorated or becoming more relaxed. Choose the appropriate routine and practice it regularly.

Your Morning Routine

The sun salutation is performed at the opening of many yoga routines, by people at all levels. It limbers the whole body by carefully applying the pose-counterpose principle: for every bend forward there is a bend backward. In this way, the sun salutation brings about greater flexibility, strength, and tone. This time-honored routine can be practiced in the morning, to awaken stiff muscles and prepare you for the day.

Begin with the Sun Salutation

The sun salutation is a good place to begin yoga practice. Combine this routine with the series in the next chapter for a complete beginner routine. Contrary to what you might expect, flexibility improves best when movements are gentle and slow. If you try to force a stretch before you are ready, you will impede your progress, so don't push beyond what is comfortable.

Breathing combined with movements helps develop control as it expands breathing capabilities. Deliberately coordinating breathing with each move will gradually increase your lung capacity. Don't force yourself to take deep breaths, just breathe normally, allowing yourself to inhale and exhale more deeply when it feels natural. Be patient and persistent for the best results.

Keep your mind focused on your movements and your breathing. Relax any unnecessary tensions, to allow the energy to flow freely, without obstruction. With breath and movement united, you will maximize the flow of energy, invigorating your entire body!

The Importance of Warming Up and Warming Down

Before you begin your routine, always warm up your body. Easing into the yoga session will help you to safely achieve the best possible results. Warming down at the end of the routine is also important. You might feel tempted to neglect the warm-down period, but this is essential. Without a warm-down, your body may tighten up. A yoga session should end with relaxation and meditation. Follow the instructions for each routine.

Begin by performing some limbering exercises. The limbering routine is found in chapter 8. Be sure to include neck warmups, shoulder rolls, twists, forward bend, back bend, and leg swings. This should take a few minutes. Ease into the warmup exercises. Never force them. Keep your attention focused on what you are doing, so that you can feel how far to twist or move. Once your body feels limbered and relaxed, begin performing the sun salutation.

Instructions for the Sun Salutation

The sun salutation is performed in slow, continuous motion. You can repeat the entire series several times, up to ten times each day, but two to three times is usual, especially if you do it daily.

Breathing should be coordinated with each move in the following way: Breathe in when you stretch back or arch. Breathe out when you bend forward or contract inwards. Make your breaths and your movements slow and continuous. As you learn to keep your attention on what you are doing and your breathing synchronized with your movements, you will experience a union of mind and body that can be uplifting. Allow yourself to enjoy this experience.

Opening position (see Figure 14-1): Begin by standing straight, with your feet together, chest lifted, shoulders square, and neck lengthened. Bend your elbows and hold the palms of your hands together, thumbs touching, at the center of your chest. Keep your weight evenly distributed between your two feet. Close your eyes and breathe in and out several times, centering yourself in your body experience in the moment.

Upright arch (see Figure 14-2): Open your eyes and inhale as you stretch your arms up over your head, palms facing each other. Arch back as you push your hips out, keeping your legs straight. Gently relax your neck back. Try to arch from your upper back, rather than the lower back. Arch slowly and carefully.

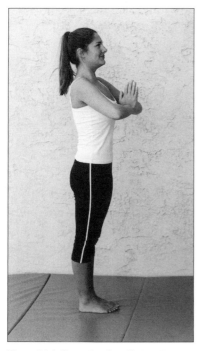

Figure 14-1: Sun salutation, first part

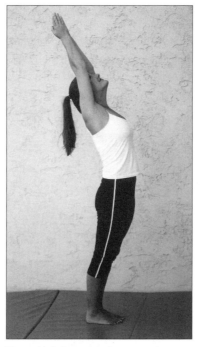

Figure 14-2: Sun salutation, second part

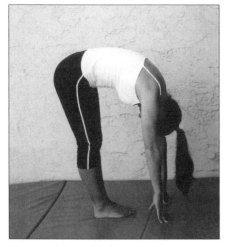

Figure 14-3: Sun salutation, third part

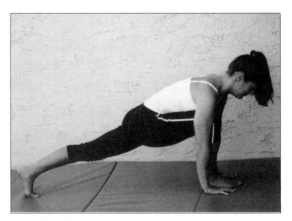

Figure 14-4: Sun salutation, fourth part

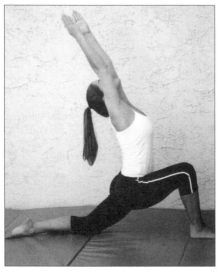

Figure 14-5: Sun salutation, fifth part

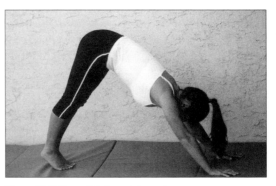

Figure 14-6: Sun salutation, sixth part

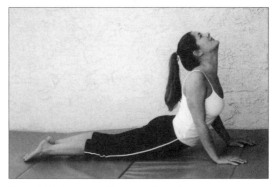

Figure 14-7: Sun salutation, seventh part

Forward bend (Figure 14-3): Next, exhale as you slowly bend forward, keeping your arms extended. Move your arms and upper body downward, bending at the waist, toward the floor. Keep your back straight for as long as possible as you go down. Let your neck relax and your head hang down. Bring your fingertips down to the floor, bending your knees slightly if needed. Hold briefly as you relax fully into the forward stretch.

Lunging arch (Figures 14-4 and 14-5): Inhale as you extend your left leg back approximately four feet behind your right. Your right foot rests flat on the floor with your knee bent. Let your hands rest on the floor at your sides to steady this motion. Then, raise your arms up overhead, arch your back and look up toward the sun. Allow your left knee to rest on the floor for balance. If you feel shaky in your balance, keep your hands on the floor at your sides as you arch. Hold briefly, allowing your upper body to stretch backward as much as is comfortable.

Dog pose (Figure 14-6): Exhaling, bring your right foot back next to the left and perform the dog pose. Lift your hips up as high as you can, as you place your hands, palms down on the floor, extended out in front of you. Expand your chest as you relax your neck and look down between your hands. Push your heels toward the floor and feel a gentle stretch.

Cobra stretch (Figure 14-7): Next, lower yourself face down to the floor and inhale as you perform the cobra pose, arching and drawing the upper body slowly up, vertebra by vertebra, beginning at your lower back and moving upward. As you get to the neck area, allow your head to arch back slowly until you achieve a full upper-body stretch. Refer to chapter 10 for a complete description of the cobra asana.

Now you are halfway through the series of movements. The second half of the sun salutation is to repeat all the same motions in reverse order on the opposite side of your body. Following the cobra pose, perform the dog pose as you exhale. Then lunge back with your right leg as you inhale and smoothly arch back with your upper body. Exhale as you bring your left leg back to your right, and lift your hips up as you bend your upper body down, bringing your head toward your knees. Straighten your upper body up, and lift your arms overhead to stretch backward as you inhale. End as you began, with your arms returning to the position at your chest, palms and thumbs touching. Pause, close your eyes, and pay attention to your feelings as you sense the effects of the sun salutation. Meditate for a moment in this position, and then begin again.

Breathing

After you finish the sun salutation, perform two to five minutes of pranayama breathing. Start with some complete breaths in a standing position. When you perform the complete breath, remember to remain relaxed throughout. Breathe in through your nose and let the air move all the way down, expanding your abdomen, then contract and let it out again. Detailed instructions for the complete breath are found in chapter 12.

Next kneel in the pelvic pose. If this position is uncomfortable, try placing a thin pillow on the backs of your legs and sit down on it. Or you can use the easy pose, or sit in a chair, instead. As you inhale through your nose, raise your ribcage and arch your back slightly while you allow the air to move down through your nose and into your lungs. Then, as you exhale, round your back slightly in the opposite direction, while tucking your head forward. Repeat the gentle movements, coordinated with your breathing, for several minutes. Remember not to force the movements or the breathing. Keep both relaxed and gradual. This pranayama exercise will help improve your performance of the sun salutation.

Meditation Topic

Pay close attention to your body. Imagine and feel energy flowing through you while you breathe with relaxed, normal breaths. Visualize your energy invigorating you all over. If you notice any areas where the flow of your energy seems blocked, perhaps you are tensing unnecessarily. Can you let go of the tension to allow your energy to flow there freely?

 Begin your day with a salutation to the sun, and you may find that you have a more positive outlook. Let the warmth and light inspire you to develop yourself to your full potential!

chapter 15
a relaxing
evening routine

By inquiring into the cause of this rigid situation binding
the mind to the individual and examining the means
of relaxing this rigidity there is great potential for an
individual to reach beyond the confines of himself.
—The Yoga Sutras of Patanjali

The Importance of Relaxation

RELAXATION IS MORE than a matter of loosening the muscles—the mind is also involved. Mind and body reflect each other: inflexible, chronically tense attitudes of the mind are reflected in the body and expressed as inflexible muscles and chronic tensions. Through yoga practice, mind and body unify with disciplined control. Relaxation of the body then leads naturally to relaxation of the mind, and the mind can be used to relax the body.

Yoga literature points to the importance of mind in bringing about relaxation. The first two sayings of the *Yoga Sutras* show how the teachings of yoga engage the mind:

> This is the teaching of yoga. (1)
> Yoga is the cessation of the turnings of thought. (2)
> (Miller 1996, p. 29)

The *Bhagavad-Gita* echoes the same theme: "He should gradually become tranquil, firmly controlling his understanding; focusing his mind on the self, he should think nothing." (Miller 1996, p. 30)

Living in the midst of uncertain times in a world filled with problems can lead to anxious feelings and stressful reactions. Yoga practice, with its integration of breathing with movement and meditation, can help to ease tensions at every level.

This relaxing and lessening of the constant flow of inner thoughts comes about with the practice of yoga: performing the breathing, postures, and meditation. The goal of yoga, then, is not simply to loosen and strengthen the body, but also to relax and quiet the mind, leading to outer and inner calm.

A Relaxation and Beginner Routine

This relaxation series includes mental and physical exercises. It is a soothing routine to use at the end of the day, to calm and relax yourself. Many of the fundamental yoga postures are found in this routine, so it is a good place for beginners to start. If you plan to exercise early in the day (before noon), begin with the sun salutation in chapter 14. Then follow with this routine. Make the rest periods between postures only as long as needed.

Warmups

Although this series may be done at the end of your day, it still requires that your muscles be ready. Prepare by carefully warming up your body. Use the series from chapter 8.

Asana Series

These asanas tend to be simple and straightforward, which may allow you to concentrate more easily. Perform each posture slowly, with your mind fully focused during every movement. Pay attention to the subtle differences in tension and relaxation of various muscles. Observe sensations and positioning.

Relaxation can be enhanced by setting the stage for it to happen. You might enjoy burning a mild incense or playing some soothing music quietly in the background while you perform your routine. Think about ways to create a soothing atmosphere for yourself, to help bring about an enjoyable, relaxing home session.

Notice how your breathing affects the posture. Stay fully attuned at all times, and you will derive deep benefit: From the simple comes the profound.

Mountain Pose

Begin the series by standing in the mountain pose. Keep your back straight and head upright, with eyes pointing straight ahead. Find your balance by shifting your weight slightly, forward and back, and then side to side, as described in chapter 9. Stay in this pose for several minutes, breathing comfortably in and out. Let your attention scan through your sensations and try to notice if there are any unnecessary tensions. Relax any muscles that do not need to be tight in order to stand up straight. Let go wherever possible, but keep correct tone in your muscles, for good posture.

Tree Pose

From the mountain pose it is easy to go into the tree pose. Pick a spot directly in front of you to look at, which allows you to keep your chin level and head straight. Raise your right leg and place your right foot, toes pointing down, as high on the inside of your left leg as possible while remaining in balance. Press the foot inwards against the left thigh. Turn the leg with the bent knee out at the hip, but don't let your other hip turn. When you find your stable point, exhale completely. Then raise your arms straight overhead and bring your palms together. Extend your body upward as you balance on one leg. Breathe normally and comfortably. Keep looking at your spot and maintain relaxed breathing. Let go of any unnecessary tensions while balancing gracefully. Repeat the exercise with the other leg raised.

Sun Posture: Backward and Forward Bend

If you began your routine with the sun salutation, skip this posture and move on to the triangle. Otherwise, begin standing with your feet together and arms down at your sides in the mountain pose. Exhale completely. Then begin inhaling as you circle your arms out and up above your head until your palms touch each other. Bend backward as you look up and complete your slow inhalation. Let your head drop down, and try to keep your arms level with your ears. Hold for a moment and then breathe out and in.

Breathe out slowly as you bend forward from the waist. Try to keep your back straight for as long as possible as you lower your body all the way down. Tuck you head between your arms as you exhale. Let your arms hang down at your sides. Go only as far as you can. If your legs are too tight at the backs of the knees, you may at first bend them a little for comfort. Later, you should be able to hold them straight. Hold this position and breathe comfortably in and out several times. Now slowly return to the standing position. Stand in the mountain pose for a moment, relaxing as much as possible. Breathe comfortably.

Variation

People who are recovering from injury or starting out very tight may want to try this modification of the sun posture for a gentler introduction to the sequence. Begin standing with feet shoulder width apart and arms out from your side to shoulder height and arch your back very slightly. Hold and then move your arms down to your sides and relax the shoulders. Then bend forward with your chest and bend your knees slightly. Lightly contract your stomach muscles, moving your chest forward without rounding your back. At the same time, slide your hands down onto your thighs for support and exhale. Hold and breathe for three counts and then straighten. Don't try to go any lower than halfway until you are completely at ease with this position. Repeat the backward and forward pattern several times.

Triangle Pose

Place your legs approximately two feet apart, raise your arms out sideways to shoulder height, and inhale. Slowly bend to the left, keeping your arms stretched out, and begin exhaling. As you continue to bend sideways, turn your left hand down to lightly grasp your left leg, while the right arm comes overhead until it is pointing straight up. From this position, relax your neck muscles and any other muscles that are not involved in this stretch, and breathe comfortably. Slowly straighten as you inhale again, and return to the starting position. Repeat the same motion on the other side.

Savasana Pose

Savasana is a relaxation position. Use savasana between strenuous postures in any routine. During this series, lie down in savasana as frequently as you would like. Take a few minutes to rest in this pose.

Cat's Breath

The cat's breath pose helps to relax and stretch the back and midsection, co-ordinating breathing with movement. Begin on your hands and knees. Inhale as you gently and slowly arch your back and raise your head to look upward. Feel the movement as you do it. Do not push to the point of pain. Let the air fill your lungs completely. You should get a full stretch along your entire back. Then exhale slowly and round your back carefully as you pull your stomach gently in and tuck your head down. Again, do not push to the point of pain. Repeat the entire sequence several times, moving and breathing slowly. Keep the rest of your body relaxed, such as your jaw, face, and neck, as well as your arms and legs. This requires focused attention and slow, aware movements.

Dog Pose

The dog pose gives a releasing stretch that leads into relaxation. Begin from a kneeling position. Breathe comfortably to prepare. Then, inhale as you go up on the balls of your feet and raise your lower body and hips high in the air. Bend over forward at the hips and place your hands on the floor, with your head pointing downward. Straighten your arms, with fingers spread on the floor, and arch your back slightly as you stretch forward. Your entire back will elongate naturally from this position. Hold for several breaths, in and out, and try to stretch comfortably. As in the other postures, do not tighten any muscles unnecessarily, and do not stretch to the point of pain. As you

Variation

Beginners may want to do a half downward dog using a wall for support. Stand close to a wall and place your hands shoulder width apart at a little higher than hip height. Walk your feet back away from the wall. Keep your back straight and extended. Exhale as you let your elbows bend down toward the floor, bringing your upper body closer to the wall. Then straighten your arms by pressing your hands and fingers toward the wall, pushing you away from the wall, and inhale. You will feel a gentle stretch in your back and down your legs.

continue to breathe and relax, you will probably be able to stretch a little more. Then, exhale as you slowly return to the kneeling starting position. Repetition over time will enhance your flexibility.

Savasana Pose

Rest in the savasana pose again for a few minutes. Relax all your muscles as you calm your mind.

Cobra-Locust Series

To begin with the cobra pose, lie down on your stomach with your legs together and the palms of your hands flat on the floor under your shoulders, your elbows at your sides, and your forehead resting on the floor. Breathe in and out several times, relaxing in preparation. Inhale as you raise your chin and head slowly. Let your gaze move upward as you bend your neck backward, carefully tensing. Then let your chest rise, curving your back up as you gradually raise your upper body, one vertebra at a time. Keep your hands on the floor, arms extended for support. Use your back muscles rather than pressing with your arm muscles to help lift. Keep your lower body relaxed, resting on the floor. When you get to the top, hold the position for ten to fifteen seconds as you breathe naturally. Then exhale as you reverse your motions, lowering yourself very slowly, one vertebra at a time, relaxing your neck, and finally resting your head back on the floor.

Next is the locust pose. Lie on your stomach with your arms at your sides and your hands in fists. Push against the floor with your fists as you raise both legs up as far as you can while inhaling. Hold the position as you breathe in and out for a few seconds, and then lower your legs as slowly as possible. Although you will need to push down with your fists, keep your upper body as relaxed as you can.

Crocodile Rest Pose

Rest again, this time in the crocodile pose. This pose is usually done after performing asanas that are done lying on the abdomen, such as the cobra pose or locust pose. Lie prone on the floor with your head resting on your arms. Let your body relax completely. Gently breathe in and out as you let go of any unnecessary tensions. Remain relaxed in this position until you are ready to continue the routine.

Easy Bridge Pose

This position is the easiest inverted posture, so it can be very soothing and restful. Begin by lying on your back. Bend your knees and place your feet several inches apart, flat on the floor, bringing them up as close to your hips as you can. With your arms extended down toward your feet, palms facing down, raise your hips up, tucking your chin toward your chest. Your head, neck, and shoulders should remain relaxed, resting on the floor. Hold for several seconds as you breathe in and out comfortably and try to align your whole body in position. When you feel ready, gradually lower your hips to the floor as you exhale.

Child Pose

The child pose is a good relaxing posture to perform after stretching or curving backward. Sit on your feet in the pelvic pose, kneeling position. Bend forward slowly until your head touches the floor. Allow your arms to rest comfortably at your sides with your elbows bent so that they can rest on the floor. You may need to shift or move slightly to find the most comfortable position. Adjust your breathing to a calm rhythm, and rest in this position.

Knee Squeeze and Rocking

This series rests the back and relaxes the hips. The knee squeeze can be very soothing after a yoga workout. The rocking motion relaxes the back even more deeply.

Begin the knee squeeze. Rest on your back with your arms extended over your head on the floor, and your legs extended comfortably. Inhale and then, as you begin, raise one knee, grasp below the knee, hold it, and exhale. You can also hold behind the knee if you prefer. Breathe comfortably in that position, feeling a pleasant stretch in your lower back, and then release and lie prone. Repeat with the other leg and then with both legs together. Carefully coordinate the movements with your breathing, inhaling when your arms are extended overhead, exhaling as you bring your knees in and squeeze, and then inhaling again when you release and stretch out.

Now do the rocking. When your legs are raised and held, bring your head up off the ground, raising your chin toward your knees, exhaling deeply as you squeeze, and then release. With both legs up, add a restful rocking motion to end the exercise. Rock gently, forward and backward and side to side, to lightly massage your back. Breathe comfortably as you rock, relaxing as deeply as possible.

Twist Pose

Gently stretch your back and side muscles with the twist pose. Begin in the upright stick pose and raise your left knee, placing your foot flat on the floor on the outside of your straight right knee, and inhale completely. Place your left hand palm down behind you, cross your right arm over your raised left knee, and grasp the outside of your straight knee. Gently twist your trunk to the left, and look behind you as you exhale. Breathe in and out for several breaths as you hold the position, staying in alignment. Slowly switch to the other side and repeat the gentle twisting motion, coordinated along with your breathing. Then return to center.

Yoga Mudra Pose

This posture tones as it relaxes the nervous system. You can use this pose to bring about a calm and serene feeling, tapping into the spiritual oneness unifying your own body with the universe.

To perform the yoga mudra, sit in the cross-legged position that is most comfortable for you. Place your hands behind your back, wrapping your right hand around your left. Inhale and then bring your forehead down toward the ground by bending forward smoothly from the trunk. Maintain the posture as you breathe in and out. Relax as deeply as possible. When you are ready, return to an upright sitting position as you inhale.

Pranayama

Lie down in the savasana pose for several minutes of breathing. Place your hands lightly on your abdomen and perform a complete breath. You should feel your hands rise and fall with your breathing. Review chapter 12 for complete breath instructions.

Meditation

End this routine in the savasana pose, for a deep and relaxing meditation. Although this position might seem simple, it is actually challenging to perform correctly.

Begin by tightening your feet and legs. Hold them tightly for about thirty seconds, but keep the rest of your body relaxed. After the thirty seconds have passed, let your legs and feet relax completely for one minute. Next, tense and relax each part of your body, one by one, gradually moving up. Finally, tighten your entire body and hold for one minute. Then, let go of tension as completely as you can.

Tensing and relaxing is a good way to gain control over your muscles. The contrast between tension and relaxation makes it easier to notice subtlety in your muscle tone.

As you perform this exercise, keep your attention focused on each muscle group as you scan through your body. If your attention wanders, gently bring it back to what you are doing. If you noticed that you lost your concentration as you worked on an area, repeat the effort again with more awareness.

Now fully relaxed, rest your mind and body together. Don't do anything; just enjoy the feeling of absolute calm. You may feel sensations of release, a spiritual experience of being detached from everyday worries and concerns, completely at peace. This feeling is your own, always potentially within, just waiting to be rediscovered and experienced!

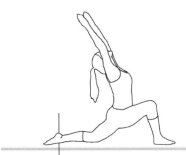

*But with proper discipline, we can make ourselves
into beings only a "little below the angels."
He who has mastered his senses is first
and foremost among men.*
—*Gandhi*

To LIVE IN ACCORD with higher nature requires strength of will and self-discipline. Commitment to yoga practice over time will result in a stronger will, along with the strength of body developed by the effort. And by strengthening the will, yoga helps practitioners to rise to the challenges of life with self-discipline.

The Anatomy of Strength Building

Yoga combines dynamic movement in and out of postures with static holding of the positions. Static holding helps to firm, tone, and strengthen. Slow-motion movements develop strength as well. Muscles become firmer while remaining flexible and subject to control by the mind. Although yoga does not build large muscle mass like weight training, muscles will become supple, stronger, and more defined from yoga practice. Two methods of strengthening are used in yoga: isometric and isotonic exercise.

Isometric exercise strengthens by pitting one muscle group against another or against an immovable object, such as the floor or wall, in a strong but motionless action. Yoga has developed isometric exercises for every part of the body, making for a good all-over strengthening routine.

Isotonic exercise puts the muscles under constant tension as they move

People often think of yoga as a way to become more flexible, but many do not realize that yoga also builds strength. In fact, flexibility and strength work together.

slowly. Weight lifting is an example of isotonic exercise. Some of the yoga asanas work in a similar way, tensing muscles along with slow movement.

You may feel the effects of this kind of yoga practice in specific muscle groups. But a more subtle strengthening, nonspecific to just one area, takes place as well. Ease into and out of slow holding asanas. Apply good sense to how long to hold a position. Don't hold beyond what is comfortable. When you feel some tightening in an area, never push yourself to pain. With practice, your strength will increase naturally, without discomfort or injury.

Building Mental Strength

We create ourselves through every action, for better or for worse. Yoga postures direct the body into a set position. To follow these patterns exactly requires action with discipline. Unifying mind and body in action with discipline carries over into daily life.

In yoga, mental and physical strength are infinitely connected: Physical strength is developed not only through asanas, but through mental focus and determination; mental strength is developed not only through meditation, but through focused attention to your physical practice. Mental strength will most certainly help you to attain physical strength, just as physical practice will help you attain mental focus.

To build your mental strength, you can use one-pointed awareness with visualization, as taught in chapter 13. This will allow for thoughtful, deliberate control of movement that will be directed to bring about positive results. Whenever you do an exercise, focus your attention fully on the area you intend to strengthen. For example, when building the shoulders and arms, direct your attention there. Feel the sensations in the muscles. Notice that as the blood flows to the area, it gets warmer. Pay attention to any other sensations. This direction of attention begins the process of unity in thought and action. Champion bodybuilders have made this a science. Use the meditations at the end of this routine to help enhance the links.

Visualization is a time-honored tool that helps in accomplishing all kinds of goals. When you create an inner image of something you are trying to achieve, you activate your inner resources by directing your mind toward that effort. Then mind and body work in harmony, leading to more effective action.

Strengthening Routine

Begin with the warmups from chapter 8. You should always begin your routine with moving stretches to ready your body. Make certain that you stretch each area carefully. Correct warmups are important for strength building. They help to prevent injury, loosening muscles and tendons, moving fluids around in the joints, while enhancing circulation in general throughout the body.

Breathing Exercise to Accompany Asanas

Breathing can help directly in strength building as you work out. Imagine that your breathing is helping to pump up the area you are exercising. As you breathe in, imagine that the air flows right to that part of your body, bringing nourishment to help this area develop. As you exhale, imagine that you are sending the toxins out from the area. Bring this image into your asana practice. Keep your attention, posture, and breathing linked.

Sun Salutation Variation

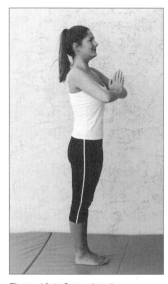

Figure 16-1: Sun salutation, first part

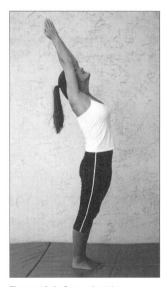

Figure 16-2: Sun salutation, second part

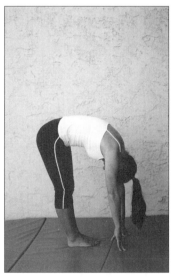

Figure 16-3: Sun salutation, third part

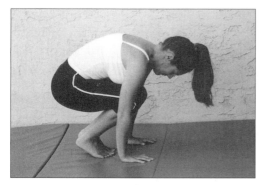

Figure 16-4: Sun salutation, fourth part

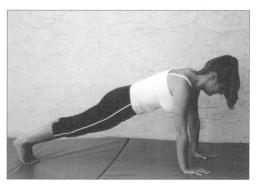

Figure 16-5: Sun salutation variation, fifth part

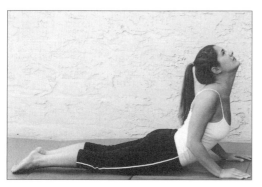

Figure 16-6: Sun salutation, sixth part

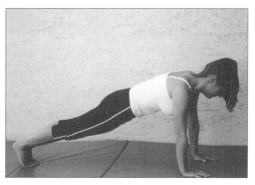

Figure 16-7: Sun salutation variation, seventh part

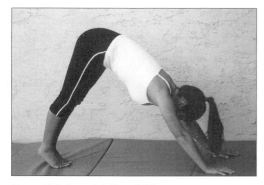

Figure 16-8: Sun salutation, eighth part

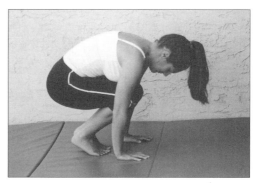

Figure 16-9: Sun salutation variation, ninth part

Begin your strengthening routine with a shortened sun salutation. For this version, make your movements slow instead of doing them quickly. Hold each position for as long as you can without straining. Breathe into the areas that are being worked on. So, for example, when you bend backward for the first stretch, feel the air move down into your lungs and let your ribcage expand. Notice your abdomen and back areas. Feel your way into the muscles. Maintain your position and breathe comfortably in and out. Let your breathing be as relaxed as possible. Easy breathing will help you to hold your posture more comfortably and to stretch even more deeply. Keep your attention focused on what you are doing.

Begin in the upright, standing position with your palms touching and eyes closed (Figure 16-1). Center yourself as you focus on your balance and breathing. Inhale as you stretch your arms up and arch back (Figure 16-2).

Exhale and bend forward, stretching your back and the backs of your legs (Figure 16-3). Hold for as long as possible, breathing in and out comfortably.

Then exhale as you bend your knees and squat down, bringing your knees to your chest (see Figure 16-4). Jump your feet back approximately four feet behind you, staying on your toes, as you place your hands on the floor to support you, as in a push-up position (see Figure 16-5). Stretch your body straight out, supporting yourself on your hands and toes as you look down. Hold this position for a few counts as you breathe normally. Then slowly lower your upper body toward the floor, but try not to actually touch the floor with your upper body. Your elbows remain bent, and arms are bent back at the shoulders. Hold again as you breathe, in and out.

Now inhale as you let your body lightly drop prone onto the floor. Rest for a moment and breathe normally. Then arch up very slowly into the cobra position, looking upward (Figure 16-6). Remember to raise your back, vertebra by vertebra, moving even more slowly than in the traditional cobra pose.

Exhale and return to the previous prone position, like a push-up (Figure 16-7). Hold again. Then move into the dog pose by raising your back and arching slightly as you extend your hands out in front of you along the floor (Figure 16-8). Give yourself a comfortable stretch and hold as you breathe in and out.

From the dog pose, bend your knees and jump your feet forward, in toward your chest, until they are between your hands, as you continue to exhale (Figure 16-9). Then straighten your legs as you fold forward, as in the third position (Figure 16-3). Your legs should be relatively straight, with head down toward your knees. Hold in the downward stretch as you breathe normally. Try to relax your muscles and stretch a little more, if comfortably possible.

Inhale as you slowly come up to full standing, lift your arms overhead, and bend backward as you look up, for a standing backward arch. Hold again and breathe in and out (Figure 16-2).

Finally, exhale and return to the original standing posture with palms touching and eyes closed as you meditate (Figure 16-1).

Go through the entire routine at this slow pace, holding each position as long as you can without straining. Eventually, the positions will become natural, as your body becomes stronger and your mind becomes more focused. This will come with practice and attention to what you feel.

Repeat the entire pattern several times, if you can do so without discomfort.

Back, Leg, and Knee Strengthening

The exercises that follow will help you strengthen your lower body. Make the movements slow and balanced. Use the support of a counter or wall if you need to. Strength develops if you practice regularly.

T-Pose

The T-pose will strengthen your legs and back while toning your abdominal areas. It also builds strength in the knees. And as a balance asana, it enhances your concentration. Do not perform the second part of this exercise (the knee bend) if you have knee problems.

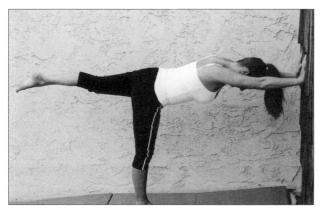

Figure 16-10: T-pose, first part

Begin doing this exercise with the support of a counter or wall if you need it. Stand upright, about three feet away from your support. Raise your arms up overhead and inhale. Bring one leg up behind you as you lower your upper body so that it is parallel with the floor. Let your extended hands rest on the support (Figure 16-10). Your body will be in the shape of a T, standing on one leg. Look at one spot on the floor as you keep your neck straight. Try to find your balance. When you feel steady enough, lift your hands slightly away from the support, to balance on your own (Figure 16-11). Breathe in and out as you hold this position, only as long as you can comfortably do so.

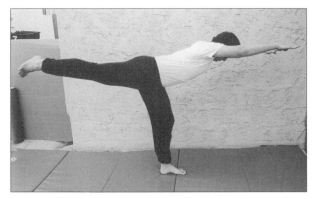

Figure 16-11: T-pose, second part

Next, bend your supporting knee as you maintain the position with hands extended in front (Figure 16-12). Keep your arms and extended leg parallel to the floor. Hold with your knee bent, and then straighten your leg again. When you feel ready, place your raised foot back on the floor, returning to the mountain pose. Stand for a moment or two in the mountain pose and rest. When you feel adequately rested, repeat on the other side.

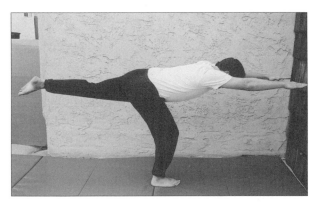

Figure 16-12: T-pose, third part

Warrior Sequence

This warrior sequence will develop the muscles in your feet, arches, calves, and thighs. It also works the abdomen and shoulders. The second and third parts of the sequence lengthen and firm the muscles of the waist and ribcage, as well as the abdominal areas.

Begin by stepping your left foot out a fairly wide distance between your legs, approximately three feet. Bend your left, front knee, keeping the lower leg perpendicular to the floor and the thigh parallel to the floor, so that the bent leg forms as close to a ninety-degree angle as possible. Keep your hips level. Spread your arms out from your sides, directly over your legs, parallel to the floor with fingers held together and pointing straight out. Turn your head to face the forward bent leg, keeping your neck and back straight. Lift your chest and stretch out through your arms and fingers (Figure 16-13). Hold the position as you breathe in and out for as long as you can without discomfort.

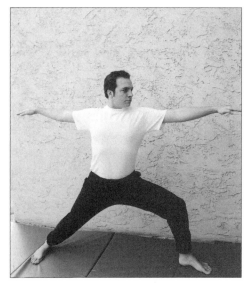

Figure 16-13: Warrior sequence, first part

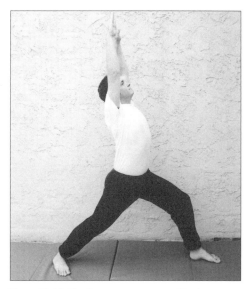

Figure 16-14: Warrior sequence, second part

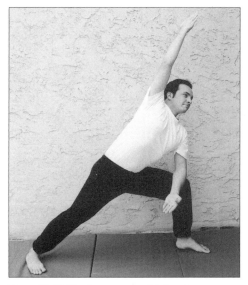

Figure 16-15: Warrior sequence, third part

Next turn your chest and torso toward the right so that your whole body faces squarely forward. You may let the back foot pivot diagonally to take strain off the knees. Then raise your arms straight over your head with palms facing forward, and arch back gently with the inhale (Figure 16-14). Hold for several seconds as you breathe comfortably in and out several times. Then lower your arms back to the first warrior position as you exhale.

Next, exhale as you lean to the right, resting the elbow of your left arm on your left knee. Extend your right hand overhead and toward the right as you lean your upper body to the right (Figure 16-15). Feel a stretch through your right arm, waist, and right leg.

Repeat all three positions on the other side. Perform the whole sequence two times. Move very slowly in and out of each position, keeping your motions smooth. Hold each position as long as you can, breathing in and out, and then move slowly into the next position.

Back Power Series

A strong supple back is the foundation for yoga power. This power series strengthens the back along with the backs of the legs. Do these asanas slowly and sustain the position as long as you can, comfortably. Increase the length of time as you become able to. Move directly from one posture to the next. Coordinate your breathing in and out as you move into and out of the position. But while maintaining the pose, breathe normally. Strive to make the holding effortless.

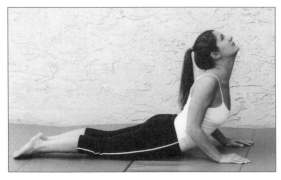

Figure 16-16: Cobra pose

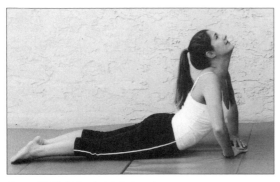

Figure 16-17: Cobra twist, first part

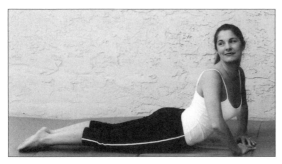

Figure 16-18: Cobra twist, second part

Cobra Pose

Lie down on your stomach with your legs together and the palms of your hands flat on the floor under your shoulders, your elbows held in close to your sides, and your forehead resting on the floor. Inhale as you raise your head up slowly. Let your gaze move upward as you stretch your neck backward into the cobra pose (Figure 16-16). When you get to the top, hold the position as you breathe in and out. Try to remain relaxed and maintain the pose as long as you can comfortably. Then exhale as you reverse your motions, lowering yourself very slowly back to the floor.

Cobra Twist

Rise again, this time placing your hands in front of your chest with your hands turned inward and fingers barely touching as you inhale. Hold and breathe in and out, keeping relaxed and focused (Figure 16-17). Lower as you exhale

People often ignore their back until they feel discomfort. But building a strong back can prevent many common back pains. We need a strong back to meet the demands of everyday life, such as lifting and carrying objects. A strong back is even important for such fundamental actions as sitting upright. A strong, supple back is central to all aspects of living.

and rest for a moment. Then, keeping your hands in the same position, rise up slowly and inhale. As you get to the top of the movement, twist your head to look over your shoulder (Figure 16-18). Hold and breathe and then lower again while exhaling. Perform the twist on the other side.

Half-Locust and Locust

Breathe in and out for a short time, and then bring your arms down close to your sides and form your hands into fists as you exhale. Inhale as you push against the floor with your fists, raising one leg for a half-locust. Lower the leg, and then raise the other leg. Finally raise both legs up as far as you can. Hold each of these three positions as you breathe in and out for as long as you can, comfortably, and then lower your legs slowly as you exhale. Try to keep control of the movement.

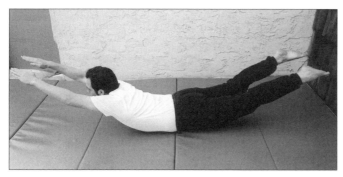

Figure 16-19: Boat pose

Boat

Breathe in and out several times as you lie flat on your stomach. Then extend your arms up over your head, resting on the floor, as you exhale. Inhale as you lift your arms, legs, and head. Look up and hold for as long as you can (Figure 16-19). Breathe in and out and then exhale as you lower your body back down and bring your arms down to your sides. Rest for a moment.

Flying Boat

Next, inhale as you raise your legs, and raise your arms straight out from your sides away from your body (Figure 16-20). Hold and breathe comfortably, then

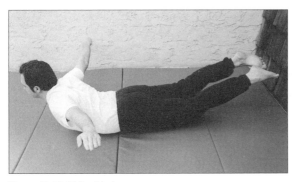

Figure 16-20: Flying boat

lower and rest. Relax and then repeat the entire series.

Abdominal Strengthening

Many people find abdominal training difficult to do. Yoga's exercises to strengthen and tone the abdomen can be just as enjoyable as any other asana. Perform these exercises regularly along with your focused attention for best results.

Leg Raise and Toe Touch

Leg raises with a toe touch will help to strengthen and firm your lower abdomen and thighs, trim your waist, and enhance circulation in the lower half of your body.

Begin lying on your back in savasana pose. Bring your legs together and let your arms rest flat on the floor, palms above your head facing up. Raise your right leg and right arm up slowly as you exhale. Keep your back and the other arm and leg flat on the floor. Let your neck and shoulders remain relaxed.

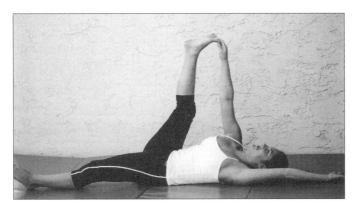

Figure 16-21: Leg raise and toe touch

Touch your fingers to your toes and hold as you breathe in and out for several breaths (Figure 16-21). Then inhale as you let your leg and arm slowly return to their original position. Do the same on the other side.

Next slowly raise both legs and both arms together, folding forward at the hips as you exhale. Touch your hands to your toes, or as close as you can, and hold a "V" position in the air for several breaths in and out. Then slowly lower back to the ground. Repeat the entire pattern, first with one leg, then the other, then both, two to three times.

Upper Body Strengthening

Building a balanced body is important for a balanced life, so yoga includes strengthening exercises for both lower and upper body. A strong upper body can help you to stand up straight and carry yourself well. Coordinate your practice of this upper body series with the lower body series.

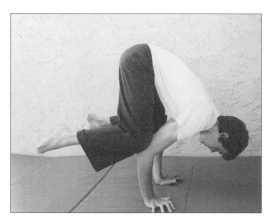

Figure 16-22: Crow and plank, first part

The Crow and Plank

These two postures strengthen the wrists, arms, and shoulders, while also improving concentration. Although they may appear difficult, these are fairly easy balancing postures.

Begin by squatting with knees bent, raised up on your toes. Place your arms between your knees, elbows bent, and hands resting flat on the floor, shoulder width apart. Let your fingers spread out like a crow's feet, slightly outward. Focus your attention on a point in front of you and inhale. Lean forward as you transfer your weight to your hands and lift your toes up. Let your knees rest on your elbows as you exhale (Figure 16-22). Then breathe as you balance as long as you can comfortably. When you feel ready, gently rock back to transfer your weight back to your feet.

Next place your hands down on the floor again and extend your legs out behind you, resting on your toes, as you inhale. Keep your body straight, like a plank of wood, and breathe comfortably, holding this position (Figure 16-23). Shift your weight to your right arm as you extend your left arm out straight in front of you, and inhale (Figure 16-24). Hold as you breathe comfortably. When you feel ready, lower your arm back down as you exhale and

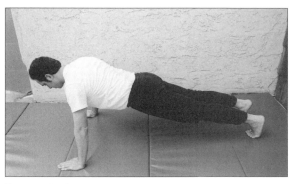

Figure 16-23: Crow and plank, second part

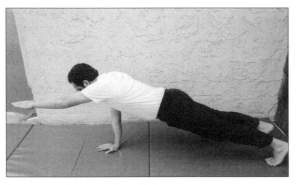

Figure 16-24: Crow and plank, third part

shift your weight to the left arm, raising the right arm straight out in front. Hold, breathe, and then lower your right arm. Hold the plank another few moments, and then slowly lower yourself to the ground and rest.

Developing Inner Strength

Adding strength in yoga is not just a matter of discipline, or building muscle. It also requires a strengthening of the spirit. The next asana will help you to discover your own inner strength.

Lion

Yoga draws from the spirit of animals to bring out the practitioner's inner strength. Each animal has a different spirit to draw from. For example, stretching like a cat adds flexibility and resiliency. The cobra's coiling ability can be translated into a stronger, more flexible spine. You can draw from the ferocity of a lion to raise your own vitality and develop the stronger side of your nature by doing the lion pose. Perform this asana with power and intensity. The lion pose helps to tone your facial muscles and release emotional tension. Following the exercise, you will feel relaxation in the face and neck areas.

The lion is performed in the pelvic pose, kneeling position. Place your hands on your knees and inhale completely. Then exhale sharply as you lean forward. At the same time, tense and separate your fingers, tense all the muscles in your face and neck, open your eyes and mouth wide, and stick out your tongue. Hold for approximately fifteen seconds, and then slowly withdraw your tongue, relax your eyes, face, and neck, relax your fingers, and settle back into the pelvic posture.

Warming Down

After a strenuous workout, it is always important to warm down.

Child pose: Perform the child pose to relax your back. Stay in position for several minutes as you try to let go of tensions. Breathe normally as you relax.

Savasana or crocodile pose: Lie down in whichever of these positions is most comfortable for you. Relax deeply as you let your body become comfortable.

Pranayama

Perform several minutes of breathing. Include the complete breath and the cleansing breath two from chapter 12. These will help to strengthen and expand your upper-body area. Let your ribcage be relaxed so that it can expand fully. During all of the breathing exercises, use your visualization skills to imagine that you are bringing in pure, clean air and expelling old, stale air.

Meditation

Close your strength-building routine with meditation. This will help you relax and also allow your mind and body to work together. You may want to use the savasana or crocodile position for your meditation, or else pick one of the seated positions. Perform any of the meditations from chapter 13. Also, try adding the meditations that follow, specifically for building physical and mental strength.

One-Pointed Awareness
Meditation for Strength Building

Close your eyes and pay close attention to a particular muscle group, for example your shoulders. Feel the sensation in your shoulders. Imagine your shoulders growing stronger. Some people will have a picture in mind. Others may feel a sensation. Keep your attention concentrated on the area. Allow your imagination to help, but keep your concentration on the one area only.

You can use this meditation while performing a posture by focusing all your attention on the area you are working on. Use a positive image to enhance your progress. Approach your strength-building routine carefully in the correct yoga way, which includes your mind, and you will gain physical strength along with mental and spiritual power.

Directed Meditation

Vivekananda offered these thoughts for meditation:

> Think that your body is firm, strong, and healthy, for it is the best
> instrument you have. Think of it as being as strong as adamantine,
> and that with the help of this body you will cross the ocean of life.
> Freedom is never to be reached by the weak; throw away all weak-
> ness. Tell your body that it is strong, tell your mind that it is strong,
> and have unbounded faith and hope in yourself.
>
> (Nikhilananda 1953, p. 591)

These affirmations are examples of self-suggestions that you can make for positive experiences and changes. Many variations are possible to extend the range of strength.

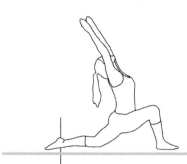

chapter 17
weight-control
exercises

Yoga may change your shape more than you think.
—*Caroline Palmer*

YOGA HAS LONG BEEN extolled for helping people to get limber for relaxation. Most people also know of its mental benefits, greater focus and deeper calm. But a new study has shown that yoga may also be just as effective for toning, shaping, and losing weight as traditional methods of burning calories, such as jogging and biking.

A preliminary study was carried out at the Human Performance Lab at Adelphi University in Garden City, New York. A group of thirteen male and female subjects went through a typical one-hour session of yoga postures, including sun salutation and many other traditional poses. Heart rate and calorie expenditure were measured as the subjects did their workout. The researchers found that subjects burned up to 540 calories during this one-hour workout. These results suggest that yoga can be an aerobic form of exercise that will aid in weight loss. An active one-hour yoga workout burns similar amounts of calories to jogging an eleven-minute mile. Note, however, that participants in this study did an active form of yoga only. Slower, calming routines

Yoga builds fitness in a number of dimensions through cardiorespiratory fitness, muscular fitness, flexibility, and a lower percent of body fat. Researchers continue to find that the regular practice of yoga contributes to a healthier lifestyle that helps people to make better choices about diet and exercise.

were not measured. What this study can tell us is that adjusting your yoga sequence for weight loss can help you to trim inches and lose pounds.

The Benefits of Yoga for Weight Loss

Weight loss takes place partly as a by-product of the mental growth and development that sincere practice of yoga brings. The yamas and niyamas, as always, offer guidelines for yoga practice, a method that brings you step-by-step to greater self-discipline. With devoted effort, you will evolve a gentle, natural approach that can be very effective in helping you to lose weight while you also tone up and become firmer. And as the body becomes more fit and the mind becomes more focused, all of these skills naturally lead to a healthy, aware adjustment to eating.

The *Vedas* describe principles for making your environment a healthy one through a program called *vastu*, which is similar to feng shui. This ancient discipline for designing living spaces shows you how to enhance the flow of prana to improve the quality of life. Vastu principles, when applied to the kitchen, may help you to institute healthy eating habits. Here are some tips:

☞ The kitchen should be free of clutter to allow an unimpeded flow of prana.

☞ Elements of the universe, earth, water, fire, air, and space should be balanced.

☞ Incorporate the most light possible, allowing it to move freely through the whole room.

Yoga Diet

"The yogi believes that the less you eat, the better you will feel, providing your food is of a high quality." (Hittleman 1969, p. 99)

Yoga offers a pathway to purification of body, mind, and spirit. Purification of the body is partly achieved through the disciplined practice of pranayama, asanas, and meditation. But purifying the body also involves care in what food and liquids are ingested every day.

Yoga has a long tradition of diet recommendations, which are rooted in the philosophy itself, as part of the niyamas and yamas. *Shauca*, the niyama of purity, is directly relevant to diet. Yoga practice requires keeping the body as pure as possible. How and what we eat is part of maintaining a healthy, pure body.

We are used to doing things in a hurry, but slowing down at key times can have positive effects. Yoga practice teaches you to move slowly and stay in touch with what you are doing during a routine. You can apply the same principles to eating. Slow down and taste your food. Chew all the way down to liquid before you swallow. Savor the experience. Dieters may be pleased to discover in the process that less can indeed be more!

Ahimsa, the yama that means non-harming, refers to doing no harm to others, but it also means that you should do no harm to yourself. Poor eating habits and bad nutrition can harm your health. Thus, acquiring healthy eating habits is an important value in yoga. Nonharming helps you to purify your body for better health.

Some fundamental yoga teachings about nutrition and diet are included here as guidelines. You may find some of these traditions helpful. Discover your own individual way. Keep in mind that people differ in their physical and psychological needs. If you plan to make a change in your diet, consult your doctor to ensure that these changes will be healthy for your body's personal needs.

Dietary Recommendations

Modern Western medicine now strongly recommends that everyone drink up to eight glasses of fresh water every day, something the traditional yoga diet has always included. Yogis add that it is important to make sure the water is pure. Drink water between meals, and sip it slowly.

Choose your foods carefully. Just as you give thought to the clothes you wear and the house you live in, you should be conscientious about the quality of food you let enter your body. Yoga encourages the eating of natural, fresh foods: fruits, vegetables, cereals, whole grains, pure fruit juices, milk, butter, cheese, legumes, nuts, seeds, honey, oils, and herb teas.

Many yoga teachers urge people to follow a vegetarian diet because yoga is against killing of any kind. However, you do not have to be a vegetarian to practice yoga. These decisions are your own to think through and make according to your needs and body type. But use moderation if you do eat meat—there is a prohibition against senseless killing.

Yoga diets recommend avoiding processed foods. This includes foods that are canned, preserved, pickled, bottled, bleached, polished, or refined. Processed foods have lost their vital energy along with natural nutrients from the processing. Yoga philosophy teaches that processed foods cannot give the nourishment needed for a healthy body. Thus, for example, white flour, refined sugar, and polished white rice should be replaced by whole grain flour, raw sugar or honey, and brown rice in your diet. When food is in the most natural state possible, people gain the best nutrition from it.

Yoga teachers also discourage the use of alcohol, cigarettes, and caffeine. They believe that these substances interfere with purification of the body. If you use any of these substances, try to do so with moderation and awareness of how they affect you. Through yoga practice you will develop more self-discipline to help you.

Moderation is the surest way to achieve lasting weight control. So whether you need to gain weight or lose it, don't try to change your stable weight too quickly. Just as you have learned to ease into and out of asanas, you should also be gradual and sensible about changing your eating habits. Consult your doctor before undertaking any change in diet.

Learn more about good nutrition, an important component of any yoga diet. Modify your personal diet to serve your needs. Many ways can bring about positive results.

How to Perform Yoga for Weight Loss

The routines in this chapter are devoted to weight loss. Supplement this chapter with chapter 16 on strengthening to tone and firm. Those who are interested in gaining weight will find this chapter helpful for trimming flabby areas, but should put more emphasis on the exercises from chapter 16 to help in building muscles.

Certain yoga asanas, when performed vigorously and with focused attention, can help with weight loss and muscle toning. A combination of dynamic motion in and out of the postures and static holding of certain positions can have beneficial results.

Increase your speed of performing gradually. Safety should always come first, and so you must be careful to keep your motions smooth. Even when doing them more quickly, pause to hold the poses. Rushing your body in and out of postures is ineffective and can lead to injury. Progress stepwise to add speed to your workouts.

It is always important to perform each movement with the correct form. Otherwise, you will not receive the benefits each asana offers. Develop a pace that allows you to remain accurate. With practice, you will be able to increase speed while maintaining good form.

Weight-Loss Routine

Begin any routine with warmup exercises. You can use the ones from chapter 8. Careful warmup of your entire body is especially important when you are going to engage in any vigorous exercise. Yoga for weight loss can be vigorous, so do not neglect your warmups!

Sun Salutation Variation for Weight Loss

Open your weight-loss asanas with a modern variation of the sun salutation that was given in chapter 16. This variation helps with weight loss as it invigorates and stretches. Its aerobic-like pace will not only add to your endurance, but will also build strength. Perform the modified sun salutation more quickly than the sun salutation found in chapter 16. Instead of performing each motion slowly and smoothly or holding a position, do each posture without pause. This sun salutation variation should be done three or four times in succession.

Begin in the upright, standing position with your palms touching and eyes closed. Center yourself as you focus on your balance and breathing. Inhale as you stretch your arms up and arch back.

Exhale and bend forward, stretching your spine and the backs of your legs. Exhale further as you bend your knees and squat down, bringing your knees to your chest, then jump your feet back approximately four feet behind you, staying on your toes as you place your hands on the floor to support you, as in a push-up position. Stretch your body straight out, supporting yourself on your hands and toes as you look down. Lower your torso toward the floor, but try not to touch your body to the floor. Your elbows should remain bent, and your arms should be bent back at the shoulders.

Now inhale as you let your body lightly drop to the floor, and arch up into the cobra pose, looking upward. Remember to raise your body smoothly and carefully, even though you are moving more quickly than in the traditional cobra.

Exhale as you return to the previous prone position, just as if performing a push-up. Now move into a dog pose by raising your torso and arching your back slightly as you extend your hands out in front of you along the floor.

From the dog pose, bend your knees and jump your feet forward, in toward your chest, until they are between your hands, as you continue to exhale. Then straighten your legs as you fold forward, as in the second position. Your legs should be relatively straight, and your head down toward your knees. All of these motions—dog pose, prone extension, jump in, and forward stretch— are performed fairly quickly while exhaling.

Inhale continuously while you slowly come up to full standing, lift your arms overhead, then bend backward and look up for a standing backward arch.

Finally, exhale while dropping your arms in front to finish in the original standing posture, with palms touching and eyes closed, as you pause for ten to twenty seconds and breathe. Repeat the entire pattern several times.

Weight Loss Series for Specific Areas

Following the all-over warmup from the sun salutation, you can train each area of the body to firm and tone. Do your workout at a steady pace. You may need to take a brief rest after doing each set of exercises. Do so whenever needed, and you will find that your endurance builds without straining. But if you overdo your exercises in the hopes of obtaining quicker results, you may be disappointed. Pushing your body's limits, before you are properly prepared, over time could lead to injury, which will put a stop to your progress. Take the gradual, careful approach, and you will grow in your capacities.

Chest and Arm Expanding and Firming Routine

Stand in mountain pose and inhale. Slowly bring your arms out straight in front of you until your fingertips touch as you exhale. Your palms face out, away from your body.

Inhale as you circle your arms around behind you at shoulder height. You will feel a stretch in your shoulders. Still inhaling, lower your hands behind you until you can clasp your fingers together, palms still facing out, away from your body.

With your hands still clasped, bend backward slightly, a few inches only, as you look up. Hold for several breaths, relaxing as much as possible (Figure 17-1).

Now exhale as you bend forward, looking downward, raising your arms as high as you comfortably can behind you (Figure 17-2). Hold for several full breaths in and out, and then slowly straighten as you unclasp your hands and bring them back to your sides, where they were when you started.

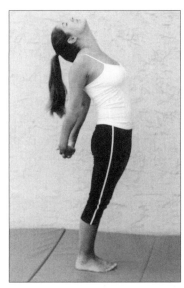

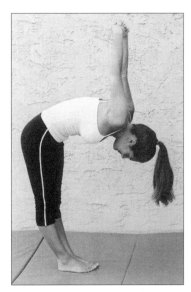

Figure 17-1: Chest and arm expanding, first part

Figure 17-2: Chest and arm expanding, second part

Trim the Waist with the Twisting Triangle

The twisting triangle trims the waist while stretching your back. Place yourself in the opening part of the triangle posture, with feet far apart. Inhale as you raise your arms extended straight out from your sides, parallel to the floor, palms facing down. Exhale as you bend forward toward your left leg, grasping the outside of your left ankle with your right hand and pointing your left hand straight up. Look at your hand and pull gently with your right hand to increase the stretch, keeping your knees relatively straight. Hold for a few seconds, then return to the standing position as you slowly inhale. Perform the same motions on the right side. Repeat the entire pattern five or six times.

Lower-Body Firming Routine

This series of postures will help to firm areas that are often difficult to exercise: lower back, buttocks, and backs of the thighs. These exercises should be performed continuously, without pausing between movements. There is no holding, just smooth, continuous motion. Make your breathing correspond with the movements.

Left-Side Leg Raise

Begin lying on your left side, with your left arm bent and your head resting

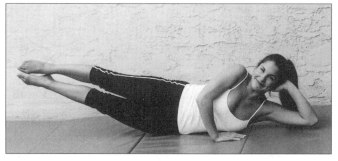

Figure 17-3: Left-side leg raise

on your left hand. Your right arm is bent in front of you, palm down, for support. Slowly push down on the floor as you raise your legs up away from the floor, as you exhale. Keep them aligned with your upper body, with toes pointed. In a continuous motion, lower your legs and inhale.

Easy Bridge

Exhale as you roll onto your back to perform an easy bridge. Place your hands palms down. Bend your knees and let your feet rest flat on the floor. Inhale as you push against the floor with your feet, raising your body off the floor. Lower your body as you exhale.

Right-Side Leg Raise

Inhale and roll gently onto your right side. Perform a double side leg raise as you exhale. Lower your legs gently and inhale.

Locust

Exhale as you move your arms down to your sides. Roll onto your stomach and form fists at your hips to perform the locust. Push down with your fists as you raise your legs up behind you. Inhale as you raise your legs. Exhale as you lower your legs.

Begin the pattern again. Repeat two to three times. After you are finished, lie flat on your stomach in the crocodile pose and let your muscles relax. Keep your attention focused on the areas you have just worked on.

Shoulder Stand and Plow

One of the accepted benefits of asanas such as the shoulder stand and plow is weight reduction. The increased circulation helps to stimulate the body. Many yoga sources claim that the shoulder stand also aids weight control by giving healthy stimulation to the thyroid and parathyroid glands (Hittleman 1969; Lidell 1983; Smith and Smith 1986; Christensen 1995). Of course, the shoulder stand should not be a substitute for medical care for thyroid problems. Remember to check with your doctor, and do not attempt these postures if you have any problems with your heart, blood pressure, or disks. You may be more comfortable if you substitute the easy bridge instead. Refer to the detailed instructions in chapter 10.

Begin with your arms extended at your sides, with your palms flat on the floor. Draw your knees up and roll forward, allowing your knees to rest on your forehead as you support your back with your hands, elbows resting on the floor. Then exhale as you slowly raise your legs straight up overhead, so that your body is in a vertical position. Breathe in and out several times and hold for approximately one minute.

Then, instead of coming out of the shoulder stand, exhale as you lower your legs down into the plow. If you can, extend your arms out behind, palms flat on the floor. Hold for twenty seconds or so as you breathe in and out, and then roll back down flat into the savasana pose to rest briefly.

Stick Pose Sequence for Abdominal Firming

This sequence combines the stick pose with the posterior stretch, both in chapter 11, for a yoga-style sit-up. Unlike the other series in this chapter, this one should be done as slowly as possible. This position contracts the abdominal region and stretches the back. It firms, trims, and tones the abdominal region.

Begin flat on your back on the floor, with your legs together and arms extended overhead, palms facing up. Inhale. Then exhale as you gradually raise yourself up, sitting up slowly while your legs remain extended and arms up overhead. Come to an upright sitting position with your legs together, straight out in front of you, back straight and head upright, hands still overhead, and continue to bend forward. Next, bring your hands down near your toes as you fold forward, gently contracting your abdomen while continuing to exhale. Then grasp and hold your toes, ankles, or legs, depending upon how far you can reach. Let your knees bend slightly if needed. Maintain this position, breathing in and out. When ready, gently straighten as you inhale, and return to the prone position. Repeat three or four times, moving slowly and continuously, up and down.

Remember that even though this series may resemble sit-ups, it should be performed in the yoga way, with slow, smooth movement that is combined with correct breathing and mental focus.

Warming Down

Fish Pose

The end of a vigorous routine includes some warm-downs. The fish pose is often practiced after the shoulder stand or plough, because it stretches these areas in the opposite direction.

Lie flat on your back with your legs straight and feet together. Place your open hands flat on the floor, just under your thighs, thus raising your lower body slightly off the ground. Breathe comfortably for a few moments and then, inhaling as you press down with your elbows, arch your back and rest the top of your head on the floor (see Figure 10-8). Try to keep your elbows as close together as possible. Breathe, keeping your torso and lower body relaxed. When you feel ready, gently lift your head and lower your body back down.

Child Pose

The child pose is a good relaxing posture to perform after stretching the spine backward, as in the fish pose. Sit on your feet in the pelvic pose, kneeling position. Bend forward slowly until your head touches the floor. Allow your arms to rest comfortably at your sides with your elbows bent, so that they can rest on the floor. Relax your breathing and stay in this position for a minute or so. Try to let all your muscles relax.

Savasana or Crocodile

Finish your asanas with either the savasana pose or the crocodile pose, whichever is more comfortable for you. Remain lying prone for a few minutes, relaxing deeply.

Pranayama

Follow the warm-downs with several minutes of pranayama. Use any of the breathing exercises from chapter 12, including the complete breath.

Meditation and the Mind in Weight Control

Food intake and exercise are only part of weight control. Mind is also always a component, playing an important role in how people eat. Everyone needs to eat in order to survive, but sometimes people lose touch with their appetite.

They may be deceived into thinking they want more or less than they really need, resulting in eating too much or too little.

Yoga unites body with mind. The unification of body with mind leads to heightened awareness that carries over to all aspects of living. You learn to pay attention to your body when doing asanas, so you can know when a tension or stretch is too much or not enough. This ability to be aware of your body's needs can be applied to eating habits as well. Practicing awareness when eating gives you the ability to sense when you have had enough. And when you eat with awareness, you also gain deeper enjoyment and subsequent satisfaction from the food you consume, while eating the correct amount of food to sustain a healthy body.

Exercise in Eating Awareness

Approach a meal as you would the practice of asanas. Before you begin to eat, perform pranayama. Sit upright in your chair and relax. Pay close attention to the food on your plate. Notice what it looks like, and smell the aromas. Pay close attention as you chew your food and swallow it. Taste each bite as you eat slowly, without rushing. Chew your food completely down to liquid. Eat only what you need. Try to be aware of when you have had enough, and stop when you have reached that point.

Meditation Topic

A yogi named Mother Anandamayi said that discouragement is the only real problem for a yoga practitioner. Anything else, even breaking a discipline, can be corrected. Think about this. Can you adopt a hopeful, positive attitude even when you falter on your diet or miss a workout? Accept yourself as you are, and then try to make improvements.

Meditation of Choice

End your session with a meditation of your own choice. Spend several minutes in meditation, allowing your thoughts to clear and your body to relax.

chapter 18
flexibility exercises

The signs of progress on the path of Yoga are health, a sense of physical lightness, steadiness, clearness of countenance, and a beautiful voice, sweetness of odour of the body and freedom from craving. He has a balanced, serene, and tranquil mind.
—B. K. S. Iyengar

ONE OF THE MOST important benefits of yoga is the way it limbers the body. Flexibility is achieved gently and gradually by easing into each position, holding it, and then carefully releasing. According to yoga theory slow stretching and holding of muscles and ligaments allows them to let go naturally.

Science is coming to accept a similar idea about the benefits of slow and gentle stretching. As scientists learn more about the body, they are encouraging people to stretch slowly and carefully. The American Academy of Orthopedic Surgeons (1991) discourages bouncing or forcing stretches, and prescribes slow stretching as superior. When people take time to ease into a stretch, they have an opportunity to become aware of their muscles and work with them. So modern sports medicine is in accord with traditional yoga theory: Stretching too far and too fast is not productive.

Listening to Your Body

Yoga practice cultivates the wisdom of the body. Thus it makes sense to listen to what your body tells you. Learn to interpret your body's signals, and use them to guide you. You will know how far to stretch by the sensations you experience as you move into, hold, and move out of poses. For example, the day after too vigorous a yoga session, your body might feel sore and even seem less limber. This tells you to be more careful at the next yoga session, and to listen sensitively during the workout to your body's communications. So continue to meditate on your body sensations, and stay focused as you move.

There are day-to-day rhythms in flexibility and tightness, as well as subtle differences throughout the day. Some people feel looser early in the morning, while others find that evening is the time when they are most flexible. Take your rhythms into account. You will have more success if you stretch when you tend naturally to be looser. Keep a journal to help you get to know your rhythms.

Stretch daily if possible. The muscles will let go of their habitual excess tension when properly stretched on a regular basis. You are never too young or too old to cultivate flexibility. Everyone needs to stretch!

As people age, they notice stiffness that wasn't there before. If you learn to listen to your body, you will recognize which areas need some extra time devoted to gently stretching and strengthening, thereby slowing the aging process.

Static and Dynamic

Yoga uses both dynamic and static stretching. Dynamic stretching takes place during movement into and out of the posture. Static stretching takes place when a posture is held without moving.

The beginning phase of dynamic stretching will prepare the body correctly for the posture. Movements should be slow and smooth, without jerks or bounces.

Once in position, hold the posture while breathing normally. Notice how your muscles feel. Breathe into the part you are stretching, and notice whether there is any latitude to stretch a little deeper. If you sense that you could stretch a bit more, gently try it without forcing. Or if you need to, stretch less. Start where you are. Your own body is the foundation of your practice.

When it is time to come out of the posture, move dynamically again, slowly and smoothly. The end is just as important as the beginning, so don't rush through the final phase. Return to standing, sitting, or lying down, and meditate for a moment, continuing your focus of attention on your sensations. Sensitive, careful stretching is the surest path to a more flexible, healthy body.

Warmups

Begin your flexibility routine with careful warmup exercises. Refer to chapter 8 for a warmup sequence, but add a few repetitions to each exercise. Careful warming up and warming down are particularly important for enhancing flexibility.

Posture Routines

Begin with the sun salutation from chapter 14. Follow the instructions and perform this routine slowly and smoothly two or three times.

Upper-Body Stretching Routine

Stand upright in the mountain pose and relax for a few minutes, breathing comfortably. Then bring your hands out in front of you, with palms facing outward at chest level, and exhale. Slowly bring your hands around to the back to give your chest a gentle stretch as you inhale. Then raise your hands overhead and bend back gently (Figure 18-1). Hold again as you breathe. Next, lower your arms behind you as you bend backward and inhale, looking up and letting your head curve back (Figure 18-2). Hold again as you breathe. Then slowly and gently bend forward as you raise your arms up behind you

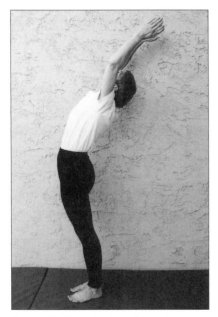

Figure 18-1: Upper-body stretch, first part

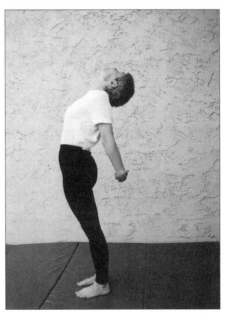

Figure 18-2: Upper-body stretch, second part

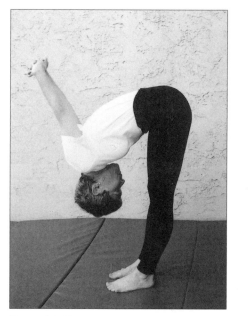

Figure 18-3: Upper-body stretch, third part

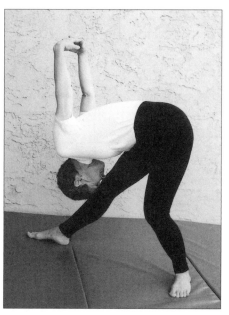

Figure 18-4: Upper-body stretch, fourth part

and exhale (Figure 18-3). Hold while breathing normally. Then, return to the mountain pose, standing straight with hands resting at your sides.

Now step forward with your right foot and repeat the entire pattern. When bending forward, try to bring your head down to the knee of your extended leg (Figure 18-4). Come back to the mountain pose and repeat with the other leg forward.

Lower-Body Flexibility Routine

These balance poses will add flexibility and strength to your legs and hips. They will also add poise and yogis believe that they can help us to focus more fully.

Tree Pose

Begin with the tree pose. To perform this position, pick a spot directly in front of you to look at, which allows you to keep your head straight. Raise your right leg and place your right foot, toes pointing down, as high on the inside of your left leg as possible. Press the foot inwards against the left thigh. When you find your stability, exhale completely. Then raise your arms straight overhead, bring your palms together, and balance. Bring your leg down and return to the mountain pose.

Dancer Pose

From the mountain pose, looking straight ahead, bend your right leg at the knee so that your right foot is directly behind you, and grasp your right foot or ankle with your right hand. Gently pull up and back without straining, as you inhale. Stretch upwards with your left hand, keeping your back straight and aligned. Hold carefully in this balancing position. Then exhale and release, returning to the mountain pose.

Angled Dancer Pose

Go into the dancer pose again. As you look straight ahead, slowly lower your upper body somewhat, to an angle of forty-five degrees, and extend your left arm straight out in front of you, parallel to the floor with your palm facing down (Figure 18-5). Hold as you breathe, and then return to the mountain pose, relaxing as you breathe fully. Perform the two dancer poses on the other side.

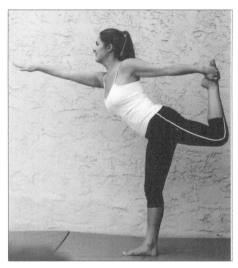

Figure 18-5: Angled dancer pose

Midsection Flexibility Routine

A flexible midsection will complement abdominal and back strength training. Keep this area supple with regular practice of this routine.

Posterior Stretch Pose

Begin seated with your legs together in stick posture. Raise your hands above your head, inhale completely, and then begin exhaling as you bend forward, gently contracting your abdomen, and slowly bring your hands down near your toes. Hold the big toe of each foot or hold your ankles or shins if that is as far as you can reach. Make sure that you keep your back straight as you bend forward. Don't round over from the middle of your spine. Breathe in and out for several breaths while you hold the position, relaxing a little more with each breath. If you can extend a little bit further without discomfort, do so. If not, do not push past this point. When ready, slowly straighten as you inhale.

Overhead Forward Legs Wide

Separate your legs and raise your hands straight up overhead. Then slowly bend forward over the center, bringing your hands down toward the floor directly in front of you (Figure 18-6). Keep your back as straight as you can, bending from the waist. Hold at the bottom and breathe, relaxing more with each breath. Extend further if you can, but again, back off from the point of pain. Then when ready, slowly straighten up as you inhale.

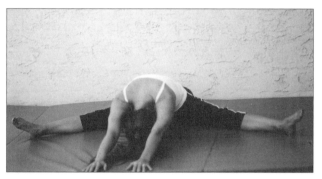
Figure 18-6: Overhead forward legs wide

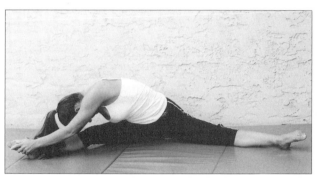
Figure 18-7: Overhead sideways legs wide

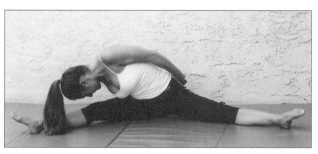
Figure 18-8: Alternate sideways legs wide

Overhead Sideways Legs Wide

Raise your arms up overhead and exhale as you lower your upper body over your left leg, keeping your back straight as long as possible, bending from the waist (Figure 18-7). Bring your hands to rest as far down your leg as is comfortable. If you need to bend your leg slightly for comfort, do so. Hold at the bottom and breathe, and then slowly straighten up as you inhale.

Alternate Sideways Legs Wide

Bring your arms around behind your back and clasp your hands together as you slowly move forward over one leg (Figure 18-8). Hold at the bottom of your stretch and breathe. Repeat over the other leg.

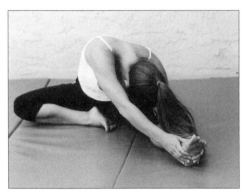

Fifure 18-9: Head to knee pose

Head to Knee Pose

Bend your left leg and press your left foot lightly against your right thigh, in a half-auspicious pose. Your right leg should remain straight out to the side. Then raise your hands overhead, with palms facing each other, and inhale. Bend forward from the base of the spine, folding over your extended right leg as you exhale. Clasp your foot, ankle, or leg and hold as you breathe deeply in this position (Figure 18-9). You may bend the extended leg slightly at the knee, at first, if this pose is painful. Later, you will be able to straighten it. When ready, inhale as you slowly sit up straight again.

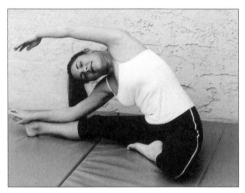

Fifure 18-10: Twisting sideways over head

Twisting Sideways over Head

Raise both hands overhead and then bring them down over your right leg. Twist your upper body slightly so that your left arm circles around overhead and your right arm rests next to your leg (Figure 18-10). Hold as you breathe, and then inhale as you come back to sitting.

Repeat the entire sequence, performing the one-legged postures on the other side.

Back Flexibility Sequence

This sequence should follow the forward bend sequence as a counterpose. It includes back bends along with gentle stretches, to gradually limber your back area. Be exacting with these exercises, and you will see results over time.

Camel

Begin by kneeling with your legs separated, shoulder width apart. Bend back and grasp your left heel with your left hand, and grasp your right heel with your right hand. Push your hips forward as much as possible, and allow your head to tip backward. Hold for several seconds as you breathe normally. Then remove your hands from your heels as you sit up straight and relax.

Cat's Breath

Remain on your knees and bring your hands down to the floor so that you are on your hands and knees, like being on all fours. Inhale as you smoothly and carefully arch your back and raise your head to look straight in front of you. Remember not to push to the point of pain. Stretch along your entire spine. Then exhale and smoothly round your back again, not to the point of pain, as you pull your stomach in and tuck your head down. Repeat the entire sequence several times, moving and breathing slowly.

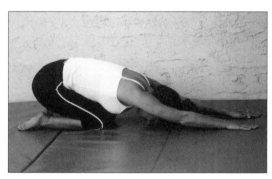

Figure 18-11: Child pose variation

Child Pose Variation

Stay in this kneeling position, with your hands down on the floor in front of you. Breathe comfortably in and out as you relax. Then inhale as you lower your head and upper body toward the floor, extending your arms and fingers out on the floor. Stretch down in front as you raise the backside of your body. Your entire back will stretch naturally from this position. Hold as you breathe in and out, relax, and then stretch a little more. Finally, exhale as you slowly return to the kneeling starting position.

Sitting Twist Sequence

Twisting to the left and right will add another dimension to your flexibility. The spinal twist series tones the spinal column and waist. Remember not to push beyond what is comfortable. You will feel how each twisting variation stretches in slightly different ways.

Twist Pose One

Begin in the upright stick pose and raise your left knee, placing your foot flat on the floor on the outside of your straight right knee, and inhale. Place your left hand palm-down behind you. Extend across your right arm and over your raised left knee, and grasp the outside of your ankle. Stay upright and aligned, gently and smoothly twist your trunk to the left, and look behind you as you exhale completely. Breathe in and out for several breaths as you hold the position. Slowly switch to the other side and repeat the gentle twisting motion, coordinating your breathing with it.

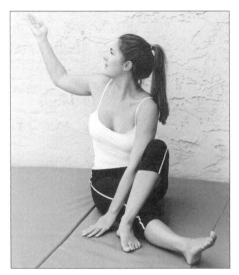

Figure 18-12 Twist pose two

Twist Pose Two

Perform the same twist, but this time extend your right arm out behind you, bent at the elbow, with palm turned upwards (Figure 18-12). This will add a slight variation at the shoulders to the upper-body twist. Breathe calmly while holding the position, as always, and stop the twist before the point of pain. Repeat on both sides.

Standing Bend and Twist Sequence

This series will add flexibility to your midsection and waist, while it also gives a stretch to the whole body.

Triangle

Stand up and place your legs several feet apart. Hold your arms straight out, palms facing downward, to perform the triangle. Slowly bend to the left, keeping your arms stretched out, and begin exhaling. Let your left hand turn down and grasp your left knee, and let your right arm come overhead, pointing straight up, as you continue to bend sideways. Slowly straighten as you inhale again and return to the starting position. Repeat the same motion on the other side, and come back to standing with arms out, palms facing down, and inhale.

Twisting Triangle

Next exhale as you bend forward toward your left leg, grasping the outside of your left ankle or leg with your right hand. Extend your left hand behind you, pointing straight up with fingers extended loosely. Look at your raised hand, and pull gently with your right hand to increase the stretch, keeping your knees straight. Hold and breathe and then return to the standing position as you slowly inhale. Repeat on the right side, exhaling slowly as you go down, and inhaling as you stand up.

Archer Pose

Now pivot your feet so that you are facing to the right, with your right foot directly in front of your left, toes pointing straight ahead, as if you were standing on a narrow balance beam. Extend your left arm out straight ahead, with the fist closed and thumb pointing up, as if holding the bow. Place your right hand on your forehead, with fingers curled in a loose fist, as if holding the string. Look straight ahead at your extended left hand and inhale. Then slowly begin exhaling as you turn toward the left, keeping your arms positioned and your gaze on your extended thumb. Twist back your upper body as far as is comfortable and hold for a few seconds. Inhale as you gently untwist to face front again. Switch position by placing the left foot forward with the left arm holding the imaginary bow extended in front, and the left arm bent. Now repeat the posture by twisting to the other side.

Yoga Mudra Pose

End your flexibility sequences with the yoga mudra pose. It will relax you as it allows you to meditate. To perform the yoga mudra, sit in whichever of the cross-legged positions is most comfortable for you. Place your hands behind your back, wrapping your right hand around your left. Inhale and then bring your forehead down toward the ground by bending forward smoothly from the trunk. Maintain the posture for several breaths and then return to a sitting position as you inhale.

Pranayama

Perform several minutes of controlled breathing. First perform three or four complete breaths. Begin by inhaling. Let your breathing passages expand. Then exhale fully, gently pushing the air out. Inhalation and exhalation performed smoothly, one following the other, make up a complete breath.

Next perform alternate nostril breathing. Yogis believe this exercise balances energy flow from the two sides of the body. Place your thumb over your right nostril and inhale, taking in air with your left nostril and allowing the air to flow down fully, as in the complete breath. Then shift your hand to lightly press the left nostril with your extended fingers and exhale through your right nostril, performing a complete exhale. Inhale fully with the right nostril and then block it so that you can exhale with the other. Alternate back and forth in this way for five to ten breath cycles. chapter 12 has detailed instructions.

Finally, do the breathing exercise to integrate body and breath. Sit comfortably on your feet with your knees together. Breathe in through your nose as you raise your ribcage and arch your back forward slightly. As you exhale, round your back slightly in the opposite direction and tuck your head forward. Repeat the gentle movements, coordinating them with your breathing, for three to five repetitions. Stay both relaxed and gradual, and you will find that over time you become more limber.

Meditations for Mental Flexibility

Meditation on Flexible Behavior

A flexible mind will enhance the flexibility you develop from the postures. This meditation comes from raja yoga. Lie down in the savasana or crocodile pose. Let your thoughts clear as you relax your body. Then think of a positive way to behave more flexibly in your everyday life. For example, if you always do something the same way every day, imagine doing it differently, perhaps the opposite way. Or if you have a troubling, inflexible relationship with someone in your life, try imagining a flexible, alternative one. Then if it seems possible, try changing the actual relationship, gently and carefully, like stretching.

Meditation on Union

Continue to relax in savasana or crocodile pose. Can you expand your limited individual self and sense your connection with the greater universe? Relax and feel the connection. Note that as you breathe in the air from your environment, you become part of the world around you in a very concrete way. Extend that sense of connection to allow your individual self to merge with the greater universe. Enjoy the experience!

part 5
making progress

As you become more comfortable with the routines, you may want to make some personal variations. Part 5 includes instructions for how to vary your routine or create your own personalized session.

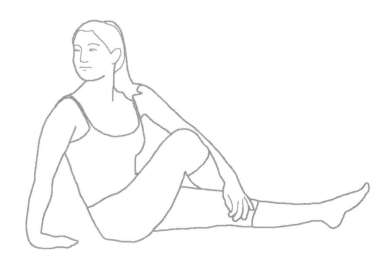

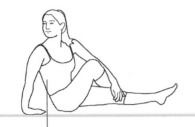

chapter 19
personalizing
your practice

*The future has yet to be made. Our present choices give a new form
even to the past so that what it means depends on what we do now.*
—Radhakrishnan

THE *YOGA SUTRAS* explain how to go about developing yoga
practice: it is not enough to simply do yoga; yoga must be
done in the correct way. Yoga practice can be personalized,
but it should be personalized correctly. The same applies to other significant
actions people take in life: they must be done well and correctly.

The first step in personalizing yoga practice is to think about goals. But setting a goal must be done with the correct intent. In the West, we think of setting goals and then going after them as the way to get things done. But in
yoga, the goal itself should not become the only focus. Too much emphasis on
secondary goals may take us away from caring about the central process itself,
which is important for ethical action. Goals
serve as aids, to point out the path—but once
you are on the correct path, let go of the goal
and instead focus on the moment-by-moment
experience. For example, when doing a posture, don't think about the result, but rather
concentrate fully on the experience as it takes
place. Awareness itself brings about profound
and lasting effects.

Your enjoyment of
yoga is one of the
key elements for contin-
uing success in your
practice. For this reason,
varying and personalizing
your routines may help
to keep you excited
about yoga as well as
aiding you in deepening
your experience.

The *Bhagavad-Gita* encourages people to
give up the fruits of their actions. This means
that people should not base their actions on

the immediate outcome. This emphasis inevitably leads to unhappiness. Personal satisfaction is not the ultimate goal:

> "Pitiful are those whose motive is the fruit (of action). . . . Having disciplined their intelligence and having abandoned the fruit born of their action, the wise are freed from bondage of birth and attain the state that is free from sorrow."
>
> (*Bhagavad-Gita* in Deutsch 1968, p. 11)

When setting a goal, broaden your view beyond the scope of narrow self-interest. One way to do this is not to be self-centered in your choices. Only then can you attain inner peace. Consider how your actions contribute to the larger world. For example, if your goal is to become healthier, do it for a greater concern than just personal health. You will have the health and well-being to make a positive contribution to others. The yoga way of action is engaged, involved, and caring, but not just for personal reward. By devoting yourself to positive yoga practice, you will not only improve yourself but also help to improve the world.

Creating Your Own Routine

Guidelines

Here are some guidelines for creating your own routine. If you keep them in mind, you will step on the correct path, as Patanjali originally envisioned for all who would practice yoga.

Before you begin your routine, always warm up your body. Follow the traditional order of warmups, breathing, postures, and meditation.

Begin with exercises that you can do comfortably and naturally. Perform each exercise carefully, without causing any discomfort, and you will find that you can progress.

Practice a pose dynamically, with flowing movement into the pose and then out of it. Once you are comfortable with doing a pose dynamically, try holding the pose statically. Gradually increase the time spent in a pose, at your own rate. Don't push yourself.

Always perform the appropriate counterpose to balance a pose or series of poses. It should work in the opposite direction for the same muscle group or area of the body.

Always breathe with your movement. Generally, in dynamic poses you should inhale when you extend or bend back, and exhale when you compress or bend forward. But there are exceptions. In static poses, breathe normally and naturally while holding, relaxing as much as possible.

Keep your attention fully focused on what you are doing. Yoga involves alert concentrated awareness. If your mind wanders away, pause or slow down, and gently bring your attention back to what you are doing. Meditation will help train you to keep your mind clear, alert, and focused.

Be sure to include rest poses during the routine. At first you may need to rest after every pose. Gradually you will find the correct rhythm for your purposes. For example, if you are trying to lose weight, you will include fewer rest pauses than if you are trying to relax and become calm.

The typical order of asanas begins with standing poses. This helps to loosen the legs and ready the body. Next come prone postures, followed by inverted poses. End with sitting or kneeling poses. At the end of the routine, perform meditation, either sitting or in savasana pose.

Consult a yoga teacher for guidance when appropriate. The extent of your contact may vary. Some people find that they can progress better when working out with other students in a class situation under a teacher. Other people prefer occasional but deeply individual guidance from a guru so that they can incorporate it into their practice. Workshops with dynamic teachers can also be valuable aids to development. Individualize your practice to suit the needs of the yoga system you practice, as well as your personal needs. A good teacher should be able to help you fulfill yourself in the manner that is best for you.

Principles

There are many valid ways to create a yoga sequence, as shown by the many styles of yoga that are practiced today. But certain classical principles have been used in routines for centuries: dynamic and static, pose-counterpose, and balance. If you know these principles, you will gain a deeper understanding of how a yoga series should be put together. Then you will be able to create your own sequences to help you safely and effectively practice yoga.

Dynamic and Static

Poses can be performed in two main ways: dynamically or statically, as you have seen throughout this book. Beginners in yoga perform asanas dynamically. This allows them to move into a pose without too much strain. Breathing is coordinated with each part of a movement. For example, exhale with forward bends and inhale with backward bends.

As students progress, they are able to hold positions longer. Advanced yogis can stay in one posture for many hours if they want to. They find the most natural position for a particular asana, letting go of tensions for the best possible stretch, twist, and the like. When you are beginning to do yoga postures, perform movements dynamically, inhaling or exhaling when appropriate, to coordinate with movement into or out of the pose. As you become more accustomed to the asanas, hold the position. Pay close attention to your body position as you breathe, letting go of any extra tension. With careful, sensitive work, you will be able to stretch a little more deeply, relax a little more fully, or hold a little more precisely in position. Thus each routine becomes an opportunity to get to know yourself better, to sense your limits and your potentials, and help you develop.

Pose-Counterpose

Yoga gently guides the body into greater strength, flexibility, and overall fitness by carefully balancing the motions together. One important principle incorporated into yoga routines is that a pose is followed by its counterpose— that is, when performing a set of poses that bend or twist in one direction, the next set of poses should balance this by bending or twisting in an opposite way.

The sun salutation is a good example of a pose-counterpose routine, bending backward and then forward in regular sequence. Another type of pose-counterpose occurs when a posture works one particular area of the body extensively and is followed by a posture that works the same area in the opposite direction. The shoulder stand and plough, for example, both exercise the back and shoulders. To counterbalance the extra strain on the back and shoulders, the shoulder stand is usually followed by postures such as the fish, which release and gently extend the shoulders and back in the opposite direction.

Balance

Balance of right and left sides is also important in yoga routines. Most people tend to favor one side over another in the everyday use of the body. For example, if we are right- or left-handed, we use the side associated with the dominant hand far more often than the other. This may lead to an imbalance between the right and left side. Some people also favor one half of their body. For example, some athletes will work out their upper bodies and neglect their lower bodies, while others will do the opposite. Yoga works to help you gradually reestablish the natural balance of your entire body. Thus, the cobra pose is usually followed by the locust pose. So when you exercise the upper body, follow by exercising the lower body.

But balance is not just physical. Mind, body, and spirit must also be in balance. Breathing exercises and meditation practice should be part of every complete yoga routine. Careful attention to breathing engages the mind and body to work together. Meditation practice brings in spiritual qualities. Over time, the postures, breathing, and meditation work together with a healthy lifestyle to bring about a complete transformation of mind, body, and spirit. Then you can use more of your potential.

Your yoga journey begins from where you are. Let it take you on a positive path for greater health, happiness, and well-being!

> Breathe as you enter into each pose
> Concentrate deeply, change flows
> Leave the unchangeable past behind
> Happiness begins now with an open mind
> —C. Alexander Simpkins

quick glimpse:
the eight limbs of yoga

First Limb: The **Yamas** are five important ways to commit yourself to abstaining from negative actions.

1. Ahimsa, don't harm anyone or anything.
2. Satya, don't lie
3. Brahmacharya, don't over indulge
4. Asteya, don't steal
5. Aparigraha, don't be greedy

Second Limb: The **Niyamas** are five important ways to commit yourself to certain positive actions.

1. Shaucha, be pure and clean in mind, body, and spirit
2. Samtosha, cultivate self-awareness
3. Tapas, practice a disciplined, healthy lifestyle
4. Svadhyaya, open yourself to learning and intellectual development
5. Isvara pranidhana, have faith in the greater spiritual universe

Third Limb: **Asanas** are the postures of Yoga. By placing your body into the asanas, you foster the process of relaxation, strength, and health

Fourth Limb: **Pranayama** is the practice of breath control to be integrated with the asanas and everyday life.

Fifth Limb: **Pratyahara** is the withdrawal of attention from the external world to turn attention to the spiritual realm within.

Sixth Limb: **Dharana** is one-pointed, focused concentration

Seventh Limb: **Dhyana** is contemplation and meditation

Eighth limb: **Samadhi** is Oneness with the universe, Enlightenment.

quick glimpse:

practice sequences

Once you're familiar with the asana sequences described in part 4, you can refer to this section for a quick and easy reference to the poses.

Sun Salutation

Practice your warmups before you begin.

1. **Mountain Pose:** Palms together in front of your chest, meditation

2. **Standing Backward Arch:** Inhale

3. **Forward Bend from Standing Position:** Exhale

4. **Lunge with Right Leg Forward:** Inhale as you move directly into the next pose

5. **Backward Arch from Lunging Position:** Continue inhaling

6. **Dog Pose:** Starting from your hands and knees, raise your torso as you exhale

7. **Cobra Pose:** Inhale as you lie prone with your hands resting under your shoulders and then raise your upper body up slowly, one vertebrae at a time

8. **Dog Pose:** Exhale

9. **Backward Arch from Lunging Position, Left Leg Forward:** Inhale as you move directly into the next pose

10. **Lunge with Left Leg Forward**

11. **Forward Bend from Standing Position:** Exhale

12. **Standing Backward Arch:** Inhale

13. **Mountain Pose:** Palms together in front of chest, meditation

14. **Breathing:** Practice several complete breaths. From pelvic pose, gently inhale and arch your back, exhale and round your back

15. **Meditation:** Visualize energy flowing and invigorating your whole body

Relaxation and Beginner Routine

Practice your warmups before you begin. Breathe in and out as you hold each pose as long as you can without discomfort. If you are trying to relax, spend an extra few minutes in each of the following: savasana pose, crocodile pose, yoga mudra pose, pranayama, and meditation.

1. **Mountain Pose**

2. **Sun Posture:** Backward and forward bend

3. **Triangle pose:** Stand with your legs shoulder width apart and extend your arms out straight from your sides at shoulder height and bend down to one side, grasping your leg as low down as comfortably possible

4. **Savasana Pose:** Relax fully and breathe comfortably for several minutes

5. **Cat's Breath:** Down on your hands and knees, gently arch your back and raise your head as you inhale, then gently lower your head and round your back as you exhale

6. **Dog Pose:** From your hands and knees, go up on your toes as you raise your torso up. Gently lower your heels to the floor as comfortable for an extra leg stretch

7. **Savasana Pose:** Lie flat on your back, arms at your sides and relax.

8. **Cobra-Locust Series**

   Cobra: Lying prone on your stomach with hands resting on the floor under your shoulders, slowly raise your upper body off the floor one vertebrae at a time

Locust: Lie on stomach with arms at sides, fists pressing onto floor and raise your legs up behind you

9. **Crocodile Rest Pose:** Lie on your stomach with head resting on your crossed arms

10. **Easy Bridge:** Lying on your back, raise your knees with feet resting flat on the floor. Raise your torso from the floor without raising your head.

11. **Child Pose:** Starting in pelvic pose, kneeling, bring head down to floor as you sit back on your legs and allow arms to rest by your sides

12. **Knee Squeeze and Rocking:** Lying on your back, raise your legs and hold in front of or behind the knees. Pull gently and rock back and forth.

13. **Sitting Twist Pose:** Seated with one knee raised, one hand holding behind your knee and other hand down behind as you twist

14. **Yoga Mudra Pose:** Sitting cross-legged, clasp hands together behind back and lean head forward toward the floor.

15. **Pranayama:** Practice several complete breaths in savasana pose with your hands resting on your abdomen

16. **Meditation:** Practice deep relaxation in savasana. Tighten and hold each muscle group for 30 seconds and then relax for 30 seconds. Tighten your whole body 30 seconds, and then relax your whole body several minutes

Strengthening Routines

Practice your warmups before your begin. Perform these strength building sequences slowly and hold each pose as long as you comfortably can. Increase the time your spend in each pose gradually as you are able.

Sun Salutation for Strength

1. **Mountain Pose:** Palms together in front of chest, meditation

2. **Standing Backward Arch:** Inhale

3. **Forward Bend from Standing Position:** Exhale

4. **Jump Down into Squat:** Keep your feet between your legs and hands on floor as you jump your feet back into the next pose

5. **Plank Pose:** Lower to the ground slowly as you breathe normally

6. **Cobra Pose:** Inhale

7. **Plank Pose:** Raise from the ground as you breathe normally

8. **Dog Pose:** Exhale

9. **Squat:** Inhale

10. **Forward Bend from Standing Position:** Exhale

11. **Standing Back Arch**: Inhale

12. **Mountain Pose:** Palms touching in front of chest, breathe and meditate

Back, Leg, and Knee Strengthening

1. **T-Pose:** Standing upright, bring one leg up behind as you raise your arms overhead and bend forward until your body is parallel with the floor

2. **T-pose with Bent Knee:** From the T-pose, bend your supporting knee, keeping your body parallel with the floor, Hold, breathe and then straighten

3. Warrior sequence (Perform on both sides)

> **Warrior Pose:** Standing with feet shoulder-width apart, extend your arms out from your sides and bend one knee and turn to face the bent knee

> **Warrior Arch:** From the warrior position, raise both hands overhead and arch back

> **Warrior Lean over One Leg, Arm Raised Overhead:** Rest your elbow on the bent knee and stretch your other hand overhead.

Power Back Series

1. **Cobra Pose:** Lying prone on your stomach with your hands resting on the floor under your shoulders, slowly raise your upper body off the floor one vertebrae at a time.

2. **Cobra with Hands Turned Inward:** Perform the cobra with your hands turned to face each other under your chest.

3. **Cobra Twist:** From the cobra hands turned inward position, raise up and twist your head to look over your shoulder. Hold and breathe then slowly straighten your head as you lower down.

4. **Half Locust:** Lie on your stomach with your arms at your sides, fists pressing onto floor. Raise one of your legs up behind you.

5. **Locust:** Lie on your stomach with arms at your sides, fists pressing onto floor. Raise both of your legs up behind you.

6. **Boat:** Lying prone on your stomach, extend your arms overhead and then raise your arms and legs simultaneously. Hold and breathe

7. **Flying Boat:** From the prone position, raise your hands out from your sides, then raise arms and legs. Hold and breathe

Abdominal Strengthening

1. **Single Leg Raise Toe Touch:** Lying prone on your back, raise one leg straight up, touch your toe, and hold

2. **Both Legs Toe Touch:** Raise both of your legs, touch your toes and hold

Upper Body Strengthening

1. **Crow Pose:** Squat with your knees bent, place your arms between your knees, elbows bent, and lean forward as you transfer your weight to your elbows and lift your toes up

2. **Plank Pose:** Place your hands down and feet extended behind, as in push-up position. Keep your body straight, breathe and hold

3. **One-Armed Plank:** Remaining in plank pose, shift your weight to one arm and extend the other one straight in front of you.

4. **Lion Pose:** Sitting in the pelvic pose on your knees, exhale, lean forward, and tense the muscles in your face, neck, and hands. Stick out your tongue and open your eyes wide

5. **Child Pose:** Starting in the pelvic pose, kneeling, bring your head down to floor as you sit back on your legs and allow your arms to rest by your sides

6. **Savasana or Crocodile:** Relax and warm down

After each of these strengthening sequences practice pranayama and meditation.

Pranayama: Complete breaths, expanding upper-body area. Visualize bringing in pure, clean air and expelling old, stale air.

Meditation: Practice one-pointed awareness to focus on muscle groups and visualize development of area. Use strength affirmations: Think of your body as strong and healthy and getting ever stronger; Reject weakness and tell your body and mind that you are strong. Have faith in yourself.

Weight-Control Exercises

Practice your warmups and then begin.

Chest and Arm Expanding and Firming

1. **Mountain Pose**

2. **Chest Expansion:** Circle your arms around at shoulder height. Keep your hands clasped behind you and bend backward. With your hands still clasped behind you, bend forward

Lower-Body Firming

1. **Left-Side Leg Raise:** Lying on your left side with head supported by your hand, perform a double leg raise

2. **Easy Bridge:** Lying on your back, raise your knees with feet resting flat on the floor. Raise your body from the floor without raising your head

3. **Right-Side Leg Raise:** Lying on your right side with head supported by your hand, perform a double leg raise

4. **Locust:** Lie on your stomach with your arms at your sides, fists pressing onto floor. Raise legs up behind you

Sun Salutation for Weight Loss

Perform these Sun Salutation movements quickly, moving from one pose to the next without pause. Repeat several times.

1. **Mountain Pose:** Palms together in front of chest, meditation

2. **Standing Backward Arch:** Inhale

3. **Forward Bend from Standing Position:** Exhale

4. **Jump Down into Squat:** Keep your feet between legs and your hands on floor as you jump your feet back into the next pose

5. **Plank Pose:** Slowly lower to the ground holding it straight as you breathe normally

6. **Cobra Pose:** Inhale as you arch your upper body up, one vertebrae at a time

7. **Plank Pose:** Raise yourself from the ground in a push-up position as you breathe normally

8. **Dog Pose:** Exhale as you raise your midsection into the air, keeping your toes and hands on the floor. Lower your heels for a leg stretch

9. **Squat:** Inhale

10. **Forward Bend from Standing Position:** Exhale

11. **Standing Back Arch:** Inhale

12. **Mountain Pose:** Palms touching in front of chest. Breathe and meditate

Shoulder Stand to Plow Sequence

1. **Shoulder Stand:** From a prone position, draw your knees up and roll forward allowing your knees to rest on your forehead. Support your back with your hands. Raise your legs straight overhead

2. **Plow Pose:** Lower your legs down into the plow. If possible, extend your arms out behind, keep your palms flat on floor

Yoga-Style Sit-ups for Abdominal Firming

Lie flat on your back with arms overhead, and slowly sit up then continue on forward until your head approaches your knees and your hands reach to feet.

Warm-Downs

1. **Fish Pose:** From savasana, bring your feet together and place your hands under your thighs. Arch your upper back slightly, letting the top of your head rest on the floor as you press down with your elbows

2. **Child Pose:** Starting in pelvic pose, bring your head down to floor as you sit back on your legs and allow your arms to rest by your sides

3. **Savasana or Crocodile**

After each sequence practice pranayama and meditation.

Pranayama: Practice complete breaths and pranayama of choice

Meditation: Meditate on the following topic: Discouragement is the only real problem for a yoga practitioner. All else can be corrected. Can you adopt a hopeful, positive attitude even when you falter? Practice eating awareness at mealtime. Begin with pranayama, sitting upright in your chair. Then pay close attention to every aspect of the meal—taste, chewing, swallowing. Eat slowly and with awareness.

Flexibility Sequences

Practice your warmups and then begin.

Upper-Body Stretching

1. **Mountain Pose**

2. **Standing Backward Arch:** Extend your arms overhead with your legs shoulder width apart

3. **Standing Backward Bend:** Extend your arms behind back and clasp your hands

4. **Standing Forward Bend:** Raise your arms overhead and behind you, clasp your hands

5. **Standing Forward Bend to Knee with One Leg Extended Forward**

6. **Mountain Pose**

Lower Body Flexibility

1. **Tree Pose:** Raise one leg up and place your foot on the opposite thigh. Raise arms overhead, palms touching

2. **Dancer Pose:** Raise your leg behind your and grasp your foot with the hand on the same side. Raise the opposite hand overhead

3. **Angled Dancer Pose:** From the dancer pose, bend forward and extend your arm in front as you raise your back leg up

Midsection Flexibility Routine

1. **Posterior Stretch Pose:** Seated from stick pose

2. **Overhead Forward Stretch:** Seated with your legs wide, your head down to center

3. **Overhead Sideways Stretch:** With your legs wide, move down to side

4. **Alternate Sideways Stretch:** With your legs wide, move down to side with your arms clasped behind back

5. **Head to Knee Pose:** Seated with one leg tucked into the half-auspicious pose, move down over your extended leg

6. **Twisting sideways Overhead**: Seated in the half-auspicious pose, twist down with both hands overhead

Back Flexibility Sequence

1. **Camel:** While kneeling bend backward, grasping your heels

2. **Cat's Breath:** On your hands and knees, arch your back and inhale, round your back and exhale

3. **Child Pose Variation:** On your knees, bring your head to the floor with your arms extended in front of you

Sitting Twist Sequence

1. **Twist Pose:** Seated with one knee raised place one hand behind your knee and other hand down behind your as you twist.

2. **Twist Pose Two:** Twist and extend an arm out behind you, bent at elbow with your palm facing up

Standing Bend and Twist for Midsection Flexibility

1. **Triangle:** Stand with your legs wide apart and your arms extended out-wards, bend sideways. Practice on both sides

2. **Twisting Triangle:** Start in the triangle pose and bend down across to your opposite side. Practice on both sides

3. **Archer Pose:** Stand with one foot in front of other, several feet apart, and simulate holding a bow and then twist. Practice on both sides

4. **Yoga Mudra Pose:** Sit cross-legged, clasp your hands together behind your back and lean head forward toward the floor

After each sequence practice pranayama and meditation.

Pranayama: Practice complete breaths, relaxing your breathing areas as much as possible. Practice nostril breathing to balance energy. Practice ribcage breathing to increase flexibility in midsection area by kneeling in the pelvic pose, arching with the inhale and rounding with the exhale

Meditation on Union: Relax in savasana or crocodile pose and feel your connection to the greater universe. Feel air coming in from the environment, connecting you to the outer universe. Expand outward

Books

Chaudhuri, Haridas and Spiegelberg, Frederic, eds. *The Integral Philosophy of Sri Aurobindo*. London: George Allen & Unwin Ltd., 1960.

Christensen, Alice. *Twenty Minute Yoga Workout*. New York: Ballantine Books, 1995.

Christensen, Alice. *The American Yoga Association's New Yoga Challenge*. Chicago: Contemporary Books, 1997.

Desikachar, T. K. V. *The Heart of Yoga: Developing a Personal Practice*. Rochester, Vermont: Inner Traditions International, 1995.

Deutsch, Eliot, trans. *The Bhagavad-Gita*. New York: Holt, Rinehart & Winston, 1968.

Devi, Indra. *Yoga for Americans*. Englewood Cliffs, New Jersey: Prentice-Hall, Inc., 1959.

Dunne, Desmond. *Yoga Made Easy*. Englewood Cliffs, New Jersey: Prentice-Hall, Inc., 1962.

Eliade, Mircea. *Yoga: Immortality and Freedom*. Princeton, New Jersey: Princeton University Press, 1973.

Hittleman, Richard. *Richard Hittleman's Yoga 28 Day Exercise Plan*. New York: Workman Publishing Company, 1969.

Hutchinson, Ronald. *Yoga, A Way of Life*. London: The Hamlyn Publishing Group Limited, 1974.

Integral Yoga Institute. www.integralyogaofnewyork.org.

Iyengar, B. K. S. *Light on Yoga*. New York: Schocken Books, 1970.

Kripalani, Krishna, ed. *All Men Are Brothers*. Ahmedabad-14, India: Navajivan Press, 1960.

Krishnamurti, J. *The First and Last Freedom*. Wheaton, Illinois: The Theosophical Publishing House, 1968.

Lidell, Lucy and Lucy Narayani. *Sivananda Companion to Yoga*. New York: Simon & Schuster, 1983.

Lutyens, Mary, ed. *The Only Revolution by J. Krishnamurti*. New York: Harper & Row, Publishers, 1970.

McDermott, Robert A., ed. *Six Pillars: Introduction to the Major Works of Sri Aurobindo*. Chambersburg, Pennsylvania: Wilson Books, 1974.

Miller, Barbara Stoler. *Yoga: Disciplines of Freedom*. Berkeley: University of California Press, 1996.

Muller, Frederich Max. *The Six Systems of Indian Philosophy*. New Delhi: Associated Publishing House, 1973.

Nikhilananda, Swami, ed. *Vivekananda: The Yogas and Other Works*. New York: Ramakrishna-Vivekananda Center, 1953.

Palmer, Caroline. "Warrior One." *Vogue Magazine*. October 2002.

Pratap, Vijayendra. *Beginning Yoga*. Philadelphia: Sky Foundation, 1987.

Ramacharaka, Yogi. *Science of Breath*. Chicago: Yogi Publication Society, 1904.

——. *A Series of Lessons in Raja Yoga*. Chicago: Yogi Publication Society, 1934.

Rieker, Hans-Ulrich. *The Yoga of Light*. Clearlake, California: The Dawn Horse Press, 1971.

Satchidananda, Swami. *Living Yoga: The Value of Yoga in Today's Life*. New York: Gordon & Breach Science Publishers, Inc., 1977.

Schilpp, Paul Arthur, ed. *The Philosophy of Sarvedpalli Radhakrishnan*. New York: Tudor Publishing Company, 1952.

Simpkins, C. Alexander and Simpkins, Annellen. "Where Does the Power Come From?" *Tae Kwon Do Times*. July 1988.

——. "Easy Does It, A Gentler, Kinder Approach to Stretching." *Inside Tae*

Kwon Do. August 1993.

——. *Principles of Meditation: Eastern Wisdom for the Western Mind.* Boston: Tuttle Publishing, 1996.

——. *Living Meditation: From Principle to Practice.* Boston: Tuttle Publishing, 1997.

——. *Meditation from Thought to Action.* Boston: Tuttle Publishing, 1998.

——. *Simple Tibetan Buddhism: A Guide to Tantric Living.* Boston: Tuttle Publishing, 2001.

Smith, Bob and Linda Bourdeau Smith. *Yoga for a New Age: A Modern Approach to Hatha Yoga.* Seattle: Smith Productions, 1986.

Tomlinson, Cybèle. *Simple Yoga.* Edison, New Jersey: Castle Books, 2002.

Wood, Ernest. *Yoga.* Baltimore: Penguin Books, 1962.

Yeats-Brown, F. *Yoga Explained.* New York: Vista House, 1958.

Periodicals

Ascent magazine
837 rue Gilford
Montreal, Quebec, H2J 1P1
Tel: 888-825-0228 or 514-499-3999
Fax:514-499-3904
www. ascentmagazine. corn

Body and Soul
New Age Publishing
42 Pleasant St.
Watertown, MA 02472
Tel: 800-782-7006 or 617-926-0200
Fax: 617-926-5021
www.bodyandsoulmag.com

Shambhala Sun
1345 Spruce St.
Boulder, CO 80302-9687
Tel: 902-422-8404 Fax: 902-423-2701
www.shambhalasun.com

Yoga International
630 Main St., Ste. 300
Honesdale, PA 18431
Tel: 570-253-4929 Fax: 570-647-1552
www.yimag.org

Yoga Journal
2054 University Ave.
Berkeley, CA 94704
Tel: (510) 841-9200
Fax:(510)644-3101
www.yogajoumal.com